10669725

Milady's Standard Cosmetology Exam Review

Catherine M. Frangie

S. C. O'Neal Library & Technology Center
J. F. Drake State Technical College
3421 Meridian Street, North
Huntsville, AL 35811

CENGAGE Learning™

Australia • Brazil • Japan • Korea • Mexico • Singapore • Spain • United Kingdom • United States

CENGAGE Learning™

Milady's Standard Cosmetology Exam Review
Catherine M. Frangie

646.7
FRA
2008
c.1

© 2008 Milady, a Part of Cengage Learning

ALL RIGHTS RESERVED. No part of this work covered by the copyright herein may be reproduced, transmitted, stored or used in any form or by any means graphic, electronic, or mechanical, including but not limited to photocopying, recording, scanning, digitizing, taping, Web distribution, information networks, or information storage and retrieval systems, except as permitted under Section 107 or 108 of the 1976 United States Copyright Act, without the prior written permission of the publisher.

For product information and technology assistance, contact us at **Cengage Learning Customer & Sales Support, 1-800-354-9706**

For permission to use material from this text or product, submit all requests online at **cengage.com/permissions**
Further permissions questions can be emailed to **permissionrequest@cengage.com**

ISBN-13: 978-1-4180-4943-0

ISBN-10: 1-4180-4943-3

Milady
Executive Woods
5 Maxwell Drive
Clifton Park, NY 12065
USA

Cengage Learning is a leading provider of customized learning solutions with office locations around the globe, including Singapore, the United Kingdom, Australia, Mexico, Brazil, and Japan. Locate your local office at: **international.cengage.com/region**

Cengage Learning products are represented in Canada by Nelson-Education, Ltd.

For your lifelong learning solutions, visit **delmar.cengage.com**

Visit our corporate website at **www.cengage.com**

Notice to the Reader
Publisher does not warrant or guarantee any of the products described herein or perform any independent analysis in connection with any of the product information contained herein. Publisher does not assume, and expressly disclaims, any obligation to obtain and include information other than that provided to it by the manufacturer. The reader is expressly warned to consider and adopt all safety precautions that might be indicated by the activities described herein and to avoid all potential hazards. By following the instructions ?contained herein, the reader willingly assumes all risks in connection with such instructions. The publisher makes no representations or warranties of any kind, including but not limited to, the warranties of fitness for particular purpose or merchantability, nor are any such representations implied with respect to the material set forth herein, and the publisher takes no responsibility with respect to such material. The publisher shall not be liable for any special, consequential, or exemplary damages resulting, in whole or part, from the readers' use of, or reliance upon, this material.

Printed in the United States of America
3 4 5 6 7 11 10 09 08

Milady's Standard Cosmetology Exam Review

Contents iii
Foreword v

Part I: Exam Review for Cosmetology

CHAPTER 1—History and Career Opportunities 1
CHAPTER 2—Life Skills 3
CHAPTER 3—Your Professional Image 5
CHAPTER 4—Communicating for Success 7
CHAPTER 5—Infection Control: Principles and Practices 9
CHAPTER 6—General Anatomy and Physiology 19
CHAPTER 7—Skin Structure and Growth 27
CHAPTER 8—Nail Structure and Growth 31
CHAPTER 9—Properties of the Hair and Scalp 35
CHAPTER 10—Basics of Chemistry 43
CHAPTER 11—Basics of Electricity 47
CHAPTER 12—Principles of Hair Design 51
CHAPTER 13—Shampooing, Rinsing, and Conditioning 55
CHAPTER 14—Haircutting 59
CHAPTER 15—Hairstyling 67
CHAPTER 16—Braiding and Braid Extensions 73
CHAPTER 17—Wigs and Hair Enhancements 77
CHAPTER 18—Chemical Texture Services 81
CHAPTER 19—Haircoloring 89
CHAPTER 20—Skin Diseases and Disorders 97
CHAPTER 21—Hair Removal 101
CHAPTER 22—Facials 105
CHAPTER 23—Facial Makeup 111
CHAPTER 24—Nail Diseases and Disorders 115
CHAPTER 25—Manicuring 119
CHAPTER 26—Pedicuring 123
CHAPTER 27—Nail Tips, Wraps, and No-Light Gels 127
CHAPTER 28—Acrylic (Methacrylate) Nails 129
CHAPTER 29—UV Gels 133
CHAPTER 30—Seeking Employment 135
CHAPTER 31—On the Job 139
CHAPTER 32—The Salon Business 143

Part II: Answers to Exam Review for Cosmetology 147

118315

Foreword

This book of exam reviews contains questions similar to those that may be found on state licensing exams for cosmetology. It employs the multiple-choice type question, which has been widely adopted and approved by the majority of state licensing boards.

Groups of questions have been arranged under major subject areas. To get the maximum advantage when using this book, it is advisable that the review of subject matter take place shortly after its classroom presentation.

This review book reflects advances in cosmetology. It attempts to keep pace with, and insure a basic understanding of, sanitation, anatomy, physiology, and salon business applicable to the professional cosmetologist, client consultation guidelines, chemical safety in the salon, and basic procedures as well as some of the more advanced and creative aspects of the profession.

The book serves as an excellent guide for the student as well as for the experienced cosmetologist. It provides a reliable standard against which professionals can measure their knowledge, understanding, and abilities.

Furthermore, these reviews will help students and professionals alike to gain a more thorough understanding of the full scope of their work as they review practical performance skills and related theory. They will increase their ability to evaluate new products and procedures and to be better qualified professionals for dealing with the needs of their clients.

Part I: Exam Review for Cosmetology

CHAPTER 1—HISTORY AND CAREER OPPORTUNITIES

1. Which of the following civilizations was the first to infuse essential oils from the leaves, bark, and blossoms of plants for use as perfumes and for purification purposes?
   a. Chinese
   b. Egyptians
   c. Romans
   d. Greeks ____

2. Archaeological studies reveal that haircutting and hairstyling were practiced in some form as early as:
   a. 1600 B.C. during the Shang Dynasty
   b. the Middle Ages
   c. 3000 B.C. in Egypt
   d. the Ice Age ____

3. The art and science of beautifying and improving the skin, nails, and hair is:
   a. neurology
   b. cosmetology
   c. nail technology
   d. dermatology ____

4. The first culture to cultivate beauty in an extravagant fashion was:
   a. the Greeks
   b. the Romans
   c. the Egyptians
   d. the Americans ____

5. In 3000 B.C. the first recorded use of a hair-coloring agent was the use of:
   a. silver
   b. copper
   c. wax
   d. henna ____

6. Hairdressing was an art during the time of the _____ for those who wore elaborate wigs and head dresses.
   a. Middle Ages
   b. Chinese
   c. Romans
   d. English ____

7. During the Middle Ages, women wore colored makeup on their:
   a. ears
   b. hands
   c. lips
   d. eyes ____

8. In ancient Rome, haircolor was used by women to indicate:
   a. personal wealth
   b. class in society
   c. marital status
   d. education level ____

9. The barber pole has its roots of origin in what profession?
   a. medicine
   b. blacksmithing
   c. education
   d. psychology

10. To achieve a look of greater intelligence during the Renaissance, women:
    a. wore highly colored lip preparations
    b. shaved their eyebrows and hairline
    c. wore elaborate, elegant clothing
    d. dyed their hair black or dark brown ____

11. A popular method of adding color to the face during the Victorian Age was to:
    a. pinch the cheeks to induce natural color
    b. wear pale shades of rouge
    c. apply brightly colored preparations to the lips
    d. wear beauty masks made of natural ingredients ____

12. In 1938, Arnold F. Willatt developed a method of permanent waving that used waving lotion with no heat called a:
    a. color wave
    b. medium wave
    c. cold wave
    d. hair wave ____

13. In 1932, Charles Revson of Revlon marketed the first:
    a. nail polish
    b. commercial hair dye
    c. mascara
    d. lipstick ____

14. In 1998, Creative Nail Design introduced the first spa:
    a. payment system
    b. haircutting system
    c. pedicure system
    d. color system ____

15. To be a successful salon manager, it is important to have:
    a. styling skills
    b. creative talent
    c. ability to manage people
    d. inventory skills ____

CHAPTER 2—LIFE SKILLS

1. Short-term goals can generally be completed in:
   a. one day
   b. one year
   c. one month
   d. one week ____

2. A personal plan that will help you decide what you want out of life is called:
   a. goal mending
   b. compass setting
   c. goal setting
   d. harmony setting ____

3. Long-term goals are measured in larger sections of time, usually:
   a. 5 to 10 years
   b. 5 to 10 months
   c. 7 to 12 months
   d. 5 to 7 minutes ____

4. Making a list of tasks to complete from most to least important is called:
   a. personality
   b. penalty
   c. prioritizing
   d. personal ____

5. The principles of good character are called:
   a. equal
   b. ethics
   c. embody
   d. enough ____

6. Using discretion means:
   a. not sharing your personal problems with clients
   b. not repeating personal information clients have shared with you
   c. both a and b
   d. neither a nor b ____

7. Being tactful means being straightforward but not:
   a. careful
   b. cautious
   c. critical
   d. clever ____

8. A combination of understanding, empathy, and acceptance is called:
   a. sensitivity
   b. several
   c. secondary
   d. support ____

9. That which propels you to do something is called:
   a. mutual respect
   b. visualization
   c. self-management
   d. motivation ____

10. An unhealthy compulsion to do things perfectly is called:
    a. perfectionism
    b. performance
    c. personal
    d. priority ____

CHAPTER 3—YOUR PROFESSIONAL IMAGE

1. When your personal appearance and conduct are in harmony with the beauty business, you project a:
   a. code of awareness
   b. work ethic
   c. personal glamour
   d. professional image ____

2. One of the most vital aspects of good grooming is careful maintenance of:
   a. wardrobe
   b. finances
   c. exercise
   d. sensitivity ____

3. The daily maintenance of cleanliness and healthfulness through certain sanitary practices is:
   a. personal creativity
   b. personal energy
   c. personal traits
   d. personal hygiene ____

4. Your clothing should always be stylish and:
   a. functional
   b. formal
   c. highly accessorized
   d. colorful ____

5. The inability to cope with a threat, real or imagined, is:
   a. relaxation
   b. personalities
   c. epidemic
   d. stress ____

6. An important aspect of professional image is:
   a. physical attractiveness
   b. physical presentation
   c. physical problems
   d. physical activity ____

7. The study of how a workplace can best be designed for comfort, safety, efficiency, and productivity is:
   a. ergonomics
   b. economy
   c. fatigue
   d. exposure ____

8. The key to prevent repetitive motion injury is to be aware of:
   a. body posture and movements
   b. ill-fitting shoes and fatigue
   c. body manipulation and stress
   d. body vascular system ____

9. Musculoskeletal disorders is a term used to describe:
   a. work-related repetitive injuries
   b. body-reducing fatigue
   c. extended periods of time
   d. varicose veins ____

10. When providing client services, it is important to keep your back:

a. elevated
b. adjusted
c. straight
d. down

CHAPTER 4—COMMUNICATING FOR SUCCESS

1. The ability to understand people is the key to:
   a. human relations
   b. operating inactively
   c. tension and misunderstanding
   d. operating effectively ____

2. You are in a better position to do your job professionally when you:
   a. pay no attention to the motives and needs of others
   b. clearly understand the motives and needs of others
   c. pay some attention to the needs of others
   d. clearly ignore the motives and needs of coworkers ____

3. Central to a stylist's success is:
   a. excellent customer service
   b. some customer service
   c. excellent coworkers
   d. ability to create conflict ____

4. The single most important communication tool that should be done prior to any client service is the:
   a. body language
   b. release statement
   c. station preparation
   d. client consultation ____

5. A form used to record information on a new client is also known as a:
   a. client questionnaire
   b. client appointment
   c. client request
   d. client recommendation ____

6. Listening to a client and then repeating in your own words what you think the client is telling you is known as:
   a. valid suggestions
   b. reflective listening
   c. reflective thinking
   d. narrow selections ____

7. To reiterate everything to a client during the consultation process means to
   a. repeat in measured, precise terms
   b. repeat in rapid, intense terms
   c. ignore the client's needs
   d. demonstrate the end results ____

8. If you experience any problems with colleagues, the best way to resolve them is to:
   a. ignore them and do not speak to them
   b. speak with them directly and privately
   c. behave disrespectfully toward them
   d. speak to coworkers about them ____

9. The individual in the salon that has the most responsibility for how the salon is run in terms of daily maintenance, operations, and client service is the:
   a. salon servicer
   b. salon manager
   c. salon client
   d. business partners ____

10. Communication can be defined as:
   a. the art of effectively sharing information between two or more people
   b. the ability to solve problems and take quick action
   c. the art of ineffectively sharing information between two or more people
   d. the ability to trick the clients into having extra services ____

11. An excellent time to discuss your progress with the salon owner or your employer is during a(n):
   a. coffee break
   b. lunch meeting
   c. employee evaluation
   d. client evaluation ____

12. In the event that a situation is beyond your control, the key to handling your reactions is to:
   a. communicate past the issue
   b. argue with the client
   c. communicate that you are unhappy
   d. ignore the client's needs ____

13. In handling a client who is dissatisfied with a service, the ultimate goal is to:
   a. argue with the client
   b. make the client happy
   c. make the client leave
   d. ask for specifics ____

14. A good customer service practice to develop if you are behind schedule is to:
   a. have the client wait in the reception area until you are available
   b. call to inform your client about the delays
   c. have the client run other errands until you are available
   d. let the client wait and be inconvenienced ____

15. To be successful, it is important for your career to:
   a. participate proactively by communicating your desires and interests
   b. be shy and not share your thoughts or questions with the salon manager
   c. be unprepared to discuss your desires and interests with the salon manager
   d. ignore positive feedback from the salon managers and coworkers ____

CHAPTER 5—INFECTION CONTROL: PRINCIPLES AND PRACTICES

1. Material Safety Data Sheets (MSDSs) are obtained from:
   a. the EPA
   b. the salon manager or owner
   c. the product manufacturer
   d. OSHA
   ____

2. Regulatory agencies and governmental health departments require businesses that serve the public to:
   a. complete a self-evaluation procedure
   b. follow prescribed sanitary precautions
   c. create individual sanitary precautions
   d. have an employee orientation procedure
   ____

3. Bacteria are very small and can only be seen with the aid of:
   a. a microscope
   b. a telescope
   c. bifocals
   d. a projector
   ____

4. One-celled microorganisms with both plant and animal characteristics are:
   a. boils
   b. bacteria
   c. decayed matter
   d. parasites
   ____

5. In the human body, nonpathogenic bacteria help metabolize food, protect against infectious microorganisms, and:
   a. prevent gastrointestinal disorders
   b. stimulate the immune response
   c. stimulate the useful functions
   d. stimulate useful secretions
   ____

6. Bacteria can exist:
   a. only on the skin or in the air
   b. only on porous surfaces
   c. only in water
   d. almost anywhere
   ____

7. A small minority of bacteria that cause disease when invading plant or animal tissue are:
   a. nonpathogenic
   b. phenols
   c. pathogenic
   d. antiseptics
   ____

8. A type of pathogenic bacteria that require living matter for growth are:
   a. phenols
   b. peroxide
   c. parasites
   d. viruses
   ____

9. Pus-forming bacteria arranged in curved lines that resemble a string of beads are:
   a. sterilization
   b. staphylococci
   c. superiority
   d. streptococci ____

10. Cocci are pathogenic bacteria that are:
   a. round-shaped
   b. rod-shaped
   c. flat-shaped
   d. spore-shaped ____

11. Bacteria that may cause strep throat or blood poisoning are:
   a. fungi
   b. spirilla
   c. bacilli
   d. streptococci ____

12. Bacteria that grow in pairs and can cause pneumonia are:
   a. diplococci
   b. diphtheria
   c. discarded
   d. toxins ____

13. Lyme disease, syphilis, or sexually transmitted diseases (STD) are caused by spiral or corkscrew-shaped bacteria called:
   a. flagella
   b. strep
   c. spirilla
   d. cocci ____

14. In humans, pathogenic bacteria are known to produce:
   a. diseases
   b. disorders
   c. spores
   d. mitosis ____

15. Bacteria that are transmitted through the air and rarely show active motility are:
   a. cocci
   b. bacilli
   c. epidemic
   d. disease ____

16. Bacilli and spirilla bacteria are both motile and use slender, hairlike extensions known as:
   a. flat
   b. flagella
   c. spores
   d. spherical ____

17. Harmless bacteria are what type of bacteria?
   a. nonpathogenic bacteria
   b. pathogenic bacteria
   c. general bacteria
   d. flagellum bacteria ____

18. In 2000, a bacteria called *Mycobacterium fortuitum furunculosis* caused a client outbreak due to the failure of the practitioner to follow proper disinfection guidelines for:
   a. sharp implements
   b. whirlpool foot spas
   c. shampoo stations
   d. styling chairs ____

19. Bacteria generally consist of an outer wall containing a liquid called:
    a. photographic
    b. photosynthesis
    c. protoplasm
    d. protons ____

20. The life cycle of bacteria has two distinct phases, the active stage and:
    a. inactive or spore-forming stage
    b. inactive and infectious stage
    c. inverted and growth stage
    d. inactive and revoked stage ____

21. The process whereby bacteria grow, reproduce, and divide into two new cells is:
    a. mitosis
    b. membranes
    c. memory
    d. marriage ____

22. Bacteria that pose little or no risk to a client in the salon setting but are dangerous in the medical setting are:
    a. daughter cells
    b. anthrax and tetanus bacilli
    c. tuberculosis and thorax
    d. acquired immunity ____

23. The presence of pus is a sign of a(n):
    a. immunity
    b. nonpathogenic organism
    c. bacterial infection
    d. epidemic ____

24. When body tissues are invaded by pathogenic bacteria, it is a sign of a(n):
    a. incision
    b. infection
    c. immunity
    d. spore ____

25. Common human bacteria transferred through skin-to-skin contact or by using unclean implements are:
    a. saprophytes
    b. spores
    c. tetanus
    d. staphylococci ____

26. When a disease spreads from one person to another, it is communicable or:
    a. contagious
    b. common
    c. corkscrew
    d. toxic ____

27. An infection, indicated by a lesion containing pus, confined to a particular part of the body is a:
    a. frequent infection
    b. local infection
    c. primary infection
    d. poisonous infection ____

28. When a disease spreads from one person to another by contact, it is:
    a. central
    b. disinfect
    c. contagious
    d. coughing

    ____

29. A submicroscopic structure capable of infecting plants and animals including bacteria is a:
    a. motility
    b. mitosis
    c. virucide
    d. virus

    ____

30. A virus can live and reproduce only by:
    a. improper use of sharp implements
    c. penetrating other cells and becoming part of them
    b. attaching to a bloodborne virus and becoming part of it
    d. poor personal hygiene

    ____

31. Hepatitis A, a bloodborne virus, is marked by an inflammation of the:
    a. liver
    b. heart
    c. kidneys
    d. skin

    ____

32. Human Immunodeficiency Virus (HIV) is the virus that causes:
    a. Intravenous Deficiency Syndrome
    b. Acquired Immune Deficiency Syndrome
    c. Acquired Immunity Syndrome
    d. Acquired Pathogenic Syndrome

    ____

33. An organism that lives on another living organism and draws its nourishment from that organism is a:
    a. parasite
    b. pathogen
    c. favus
    d. contaminant

    ____

34. If nail implements have not been disinfected properly, the client may contract:
    a. nail condition
    b. nail enhancements
    c. nail designs
    d. nail fungus

    ____

35. Disease-causing bacteria or viruses that are carried through the body in the blood or body fluids are:
    a. bloodborne pathogens
    b. bloodborne capitis
    c. bloodborne elements
    d. bloodborne scabies

    ____

36. Transmission of bloodborne pathogens can become possible through shaving, nipping, facial treatments, waxing, tweezing, or:
    a. sometimes if the skin barrier is broken
    b. anytime the skin barrier is broken
    c. when the skin is disinfected
    d. when the technician uses great care

    ____

37. A skin disease caused by an infestation of head lice is:
    a. perpendicular
    b. scabies
    c. pediculosis
    d. peroxide ____

38. The ability of the body to destroy pathogenic bacteria or viruses that have entered the body is:
    a. immunity
    b. epidemic
    c. skin lesion
    d. immigration ____

39. The type of immunity the body develops after overcoming a disease or through vaccinations is:
    a. casual contact
    b. acquired immunity
    c. acquired contact
    d. an epidemic ____

40. The surfaces of tools or objects not completely free from dirt, oils, and microbes are covered with:
    a. cholesterol
    b. containers
    c. immunization
    d. contaminants ____

41. The process of removing pathogens and other substances from tools and surfaces is:
    a. decontamination
    b. scrubbing
    c. washing
    d. cleaning ____

42. The three main types of decontamination are:
    a. disinfection, washing, and autoclave
    b. sanitation, disinfection, and sterilization
    c. sterilization, contaminants, and sanitation
    d. antiseptic, disinfection, and sterilization ____

43. Decontamination is a process that involves the use of:
    a. physical and sensitive means to remove or destroy pathogens
    b. sanitation and the use of closed containers
    c. physical or chemical means to remove or destroy pathogens
    d. antiseptic practices and autoclaves ____

44. Estheticians who use needles and probes that lance the skin must use a level of decontamination called:
    a. sterilization
    b. presterilization
    c. phenols and bleach
    d. dry heat sterilization ____

45. In the salon setting, disinfection is extremely effective in controlling:
    a. microorganisms on non-living surfaces
    b. wet sanitizers on living surfaces
    c. soap and warm water
    d. disinfection procedures ____

46. A higher level of decontamination than sanitation is:
   a. disinfection
   b. pathogenic
   c. discarded
   d. scrubbing ____

47. An exception to the level of protection that disinfection provides and the possibility of an infection could be present if:
   a. the client's skin is broken
   b. the client is washed and ready
   c. the item is given to the client
   d. the client has several services ____

48. A chemical agent that is used to destroy bacteria and viruses on surfaces is:
   a. 10% alcohol
   b. disinfectant
   c. antiseptic
   d. 20% peroxide ____

49. Disinfectants must have a registration number and be approved by the:
   a. Environmental Protection Agency (EPA)
   b. Occupation Protection Agency (OPA)
   c. U.S. Department of Labor (DOL)
   d. Food and Drug Administration (FDA) ____

50. A manufacturer must supply pertinent safety and storage information by providing:
   a. Material Storage Sheets
   b. Occupational Safety and Health
   c. Material Safety Data Sheets
   d. Material Forms and Invoices ____

51. The agency that enforces safety and health standards in the workplace is:
   a. OSHA
   b. FDA
   c. DOL
   d. EPA ____

52. A disinfectant that meets regulatory agency requirements for destroying bacteria, fungi, and viruses is:
   a. bacterial, pathogenic, and virucidal
   b. bacterial, fungicidal, and virucidal
   c. bacterial, solvent, and disinfectional
   d. HIV, fungicidal, and sporicidal ____

53. A disinfectant used in salons should be appropriate and have the correct:
   a. efficiency
   b. excellency
   c. efficacy
   d. control measures ____

54. A salon implement that accidentally comes in contact with blood or body fluids should be cleaned and:
   a. completely immersed in an EPA-registered disinfectant
   b. washed and rinsed in an EPA-registered tuberculocidal antiseptic that kills HIV and HBV
   c. washed and placed in an EPA-registered antiseptic that kills HIV and hepatitis
   d. washed and immersed in an EPA-registered solution that kills HIV and AIDS ____

55. Any Item that cannot be disinfected after use on a client must be:
   a. washed
   b. recycled
   c. reused
   d. discarded ____

56. Common, very safe, and useful types of disinfectant that contain sophisticated blends that work to disinfect implements in 10 to 15 minutes are:
   a. quaternary ammonium compounds
   b. quaternary peroxide antiseptics
   c. ammonium phenols and bleach
   d. 70% isopropyl alcohol ____

57. Disinfectant with a high pH that can cause skin irritation or burn the skin or eyes are:
   a. alcohol and bleach
   b. EPA-registered disinfectants
   c. alcohol and quats
   d. phenolic disinfectants ____

58. To be effective in the disinfection of implements, ethyl alcohol must be no less than:
   a. 20 percent
   b. 70 percent
   c. 75 percent
   d. 85 percent ____

59. A common household product used effectively as a disinfectant is:
   a. sodium hypochlorite
   b. sodium alcohol
   c. formalin
   d. sodium hydroxide ____

60. When mixing a disinfectant solution, add disinfectant to water and:
   a. mix more solution than is necessary
   b. mix equal parts of water and disinfectant solution
   c. mix according to the manufacturer's exact directions
   d. mix in sink areas to avoid spills ____

61. To avoid contaminating implements, remove from a disinfectant solution using:
    a. tongs, basket, or gloves
    b. clean hands and fingers
    c. bare fingers
    d. middle finger and thumb ____

62. Store a clean, disinfected implement in:
    a. an open container at the station
    b. a station drawer with other implements
    c. an open drawer at the front desk
    d. a clean, dry container ____

63. How often must individual towels and linens be set aside to be laundered?
    a. after use on a client
    b. at the end of the day
    c. at least once a week
    d. no less than twice a month ____

64. The contact points of equipment that cannot be immersed in liquid solutions should be cleaned and disinfected using a:
    a. regulatory oversight agency approved disinfectant
    b. regulatory oversight agency approved antiseptic
    c. solution weaker than necessary
    d. solution that does not kill bacteria ____

65. At the end of the day, the disinfection procedure for a foot spa should include removing and cleaning the screen, washing the screen and inlet with soap and water, and totally immersing the screen in an approved disinfectant according to manufacturers' directions and:
    a. flushing with water and letting air-dry till the next day
    b. flushing the system with low-sudsing soap and warm water for 10 minutes, rinsing, draining, and letting air-dry
    c. removing the clean the screen if it appears dirty
    d. removing the screen and spraying it with a disinfectant solution ____

66. Every week, foot spas should be cleaned following the daily procedure and filled with:
    a. a disinfectant solution and left for 20 minutes, then drained and flushed
    b. a 10% bleach solution and left 10 minutes, then drained and flushed
    c. a disinfectant solution and left at least 6 to 10 hours, then drained and flushed
    d. a solution of hot soapy water ____

67. Any disposable material used in cleaning blood spills should be:
   a. placed in the recycle bin with the regular trash
   b. disposed of immediately
   c. placed in double bags before disposing or placed in a container for contaminated waste
   d. left at the station area ____

68. The first step in the decontamination process is called:
   a. sanitation
   b. disinfection
   c. antiseptic cleansing
   d. surface wiping ____

69. When using liquid soap, scrub your hands and lather for at least:
   a. 5 minutes
   b. 20 seconds
   c. 1 minute
   d. 10 seconds ____

70. The use of bar soap is prohibited in most salons because bar soaps:
   a. are expensive
   b. lather too much
   c. grow bacteria
   d. lead to skin infections ____

71. Which of these is a danger of using antibacterial soaps?
   a. They often do not kill germs and bacteria on the hands.
   b. They often cause the skin to dry quickly, causing fissures.
   c. They are ineffective in removing dirt and grime from the hands.
   d. They may promote the growth of resistant strains. ____

72. Antiseptics are effective for:
   a. disinfecting instruments
   b. sanitizing the hands
   c. disinfecting equipment
   d. sterilizing equipment ____

73. The agency that sets the standard for dealing with bloodborne pathogens is:
   a. OSHA
   b. FBI
   c. MSDS
   d. FDA ____

74. Universal precautions require employees to assume that human blood and body fluids are infectious for:
   a. nonpathogenic pathogens
   b. bloodborne pathogens
   c. flu
   d. immunity ____

75. A client that is infected with Hepatitis B or other bloodborne pathogens and shows no symptoms or signs of infection is:
   a. asymptomatic
   b. not infectious
   c. healthy
   d. in remission ____

CHAPTER 6—GENERAL ANATOMY AND PHYSIOLOGY

1. Cosmetology is primarily restricted to the muscles, nerves, circulatory system, and:
   a. bones of the head, face, neck, arms, hands, lower legs, and feet
   b. bones of the legs, feet, and hands
   c. muscles and nerves of the head and face
   d. nerves and blood vessels of the hands, neck, face, and leg ____

2. The basic unit of all living things is the:
   a. anatomy
   b. cell
   c. muscle
   d. nerve ____

3. The substance called protoplasm is found in:
   a. the cells of all living things
   b. the tissues and organs
   c. the structure of the human body
   d. inanimate objects ____

4. The study of the structures of the human body is:
   a. protoplasm
   b. physiology
   c. structure
   d. anatomy ____

5. A dense active protoplasm found in the center of the cell is:
   a. density
   b. growth
   c. nucleus
   d. structure ____

6. Most cells reproduce by dividing into two identical cells called:
   a. constructive metabolism
   b. daughter cells
   c. reproductive cells
   d. building cells ____

7. The watery fluid that cells need for growth, reproduction, and self-repair is found in the:
   a. cystine
   b. anatomy
   c. cytoplasm
   d. nerve tissue ____

8. The chemical process whereby cells are nourished and carry out their activities is:
   a. metabolism
   b. mitosis
   c. membrane
   d. memory cells ____

9. The chemical process of cell nourishment has two phases, which are:
   a. anabolism and catabolism
   b. reproduction and anabolism
   c. anabolism and repair
   d. plasma and myology ____

10. A collection of similar cells that perform a specific function are:
    a. ligaments
    b. body fluids
    c. tendons
    d. tissue ____

11. A type of tissue that supports, protects, and binds together other tissues of the body is:
    a. nerve endings
    b. connective tissue
    c. coordinating tissue
    d. nerve tissue ____

12. Tissues that are a protective covering on the skin or the lining of the heart and glands are examples of:
    a. epithelial tissue
    b. epidermis tissue
    c. exit tissue
    d. specific function tissue ____

13. Nerve tissue is composed of special cells known as:
    a. respiratory tissue
    b. glands
    c. neurons
    d. tendons ____

14. The physical foundation of the body is the:
    a. circulatory system
    b. muscular system
    c. integumentary system
    d. skeletal system ____

15. The connection between two or more bones is a:
    a. tissue
    b. joint
    c. tendon
    d. muscle ____

16. The scientific name for the study of the anatomy, structure, and function of the bones is:
    a. orthopaedic
    b. osteology
    c. trichology
    d. microbiology ____

17. The ankle joint is formed by the tibia, fibula, and the:
    a. patella
    b. femur
    c. talus
    d. radius ____

18. The oval, bony case that protects the brain is the:
    a. circle
    b. facial skeleton
    c. cranium
    d. occipital bone ____

19. The hindmost bone of the skull, below the parietal bone, which forms the back of the skull above the nape is the:
    a. cranium bone
    b. occipital bone
    c. frontal bone
    d. temporal bones ____

20. The bones of the face are involved in:
    a. facial expressions
    b. facial bridges
    c. facial massage
    d. connective tissue ____

21. The system of the body that covers, shapes, and supports the skeleton tissue is the:
    a. muscular system
    b. muscular tissue
    c. respiratory system
    d. digestive system ____

22. The medical term used to describe the study, function, and diseases of the muscles is:
    a. microbiology
    b. esthetics
    c. osteology
    d. myology ____

23. The two bones that form the upper jaw are:
    a. nasal bones
    b. maxillae bones
    c. sternum bones
    d. cranium bones ____

24. The two bones that form the sides and crown (top) of the cranium are the:
    a. parietal bones
    b. occipital bones
    c. nasal bones
    d. frontal bones ____

25. The uppermost and largest bone of the arm, extending from the elbow to the shoulder, is the:
    a. carpus
    b. humerus
    c. phalanges
    d. radius ____

26. The foot is made up of _____ bones.
    a. 16
    b. 26
    c. 18
    d. 24 ____

27. The _____ is a heavy, long bone that forms the leg above the knee.
    a. fibula
    b. ulna
    c. femur
    d. talus ____

28. Muscles are fibrous tissue classified as three types, which are:
    a. buccinator, superior, and cardiac
    b. stretch, nonstretch, and cardiac
    c. cardiac, insertion, and striated
    d. striated, nonstriated, and cardiac ____

29. Skeletal muscles attached to bone that are voluntary or controlled at will are:
    a. striated muscle
    b. cardiac muscle
    c. epicranius muscle
    d. trapezius muscle ____

30. The part of the muscle that does not move is the:
    a. cardiac
    b. insertion
    c. origin
    d. tendon ____

31. Pressure applied to a muscle during a massage is usually directed from the:
    a. middle to insertion
    b. beginning to end
    c. major to minor
    d. insertion to the origin ____

32. The broad muscle that covers the top of the head is the:
    a. temporal
    b. epicranius
    c. deltoid
    d. occipital
    ____

33. The front portion of the epicranius that raises the eyebrows, draws the scalp forward, and causes wrinkles across the forehead is the:
    a. frontalis
    b. occipitalis
    c. ligament
    d. temporalis
    ____

34. The sternocleidomastoid muscle is the muscle of the neck that is responsible for:
    a. raising and lowering the eyes
    b. raising and lowering the arms
    c. lowering and rotating the head
    d. raising the mouth
    ____

35. The ring muscle of the eye socket that enables the eyes to close is the:
    a. orbicularis minor
    b. posterior muscle
    c. orbicularis oculi
    d. serratus anterior
    ____

36. A muscle covering the back of the neck and the upper and middle region of the back that rotates and controls the swinging of the arms is the:
    a. deltoid
    b. trapezius
    c. platysma
    d. zygomaticus
    ____

37. Muscles that straighten the wrist, hand, and fingers to form a straight line are the:
    a. extensors
    b. digits
    c. deltoids
    d. biceps
    ____

38. The muscles at the base of the fingers that draw fingers together are the:
    a. tendons
    b. abductors
    c. extensors
    d. adductors
    ____

39. The gastrocnemius muscle is located in the:
    a. lower leg
    b. palm of hand
    c. mouth
    d. lower arm
    ____

40. The scientific study of the structure, function, and pathology of the nervous system is:
    a. neutrons
    b. neurology
    c. myology
    d. osteology
    ____

41. Every square inch of the body is supplied with fine fibers known as:
    a. neutrons
    b. platysma
    c. nerves
    d. cells
    ____

42. The nervous system that controls the brain, spinal cord, spinal nerves, and cranial nerves is the:
    a. central nervous system
    b. voluntary nervous system
    c. peripheral nervous system
    d. spinal nervous system
    ____

43. The system of nerves that carries impulses or messages to and from the central nervous system is the:
    a. involuntary nervous system
    b. respiratory nervous system
    c. mental nerve system
    d. peripheral nervous system
    ____

44. The portion of the central nervous system that originates in the brain, extends down the lower extremity of the trunk, and is protected is the:
    a. spinal cord
    b. cell belly
    c. spinal atria
    d. nasal nerve
    ____

45. The largest and most complex nerve tissue in the body is the:
    a. axon
    b. spine
    c. heart
    d. brain
    ____

46. Whitish cords made up of bundles of nerve fibers held together by connective tissue are:
    a. neutrons
    b. nerves
    c. valves
    d. ventricles
    ____

47. Sensory nerve endings that are located close to the surface of the skin are:
    a. receptors
    b. reactions
    c. capillaries
    d. spinal nerves
    ____

48. Nerves that carry impulses from the brain to the muscles and produce movement are:
    a. median nerves
    b. motor cells
    c. spinal nerves
    d. motor nerves
    ____

49. The largest of the cranial nerves, also known as the trifacial nerve or the trigeminal nerve, is the:
    a. fourth cranial nerve
    b. fifth cranial nerve
    c. supraorbital nerve
    d. maxillary nerve
    ____

50. The chief motor nerve of the face that emerges near the lower part of the ear and extends to the muscles of the neck is the:
    a. digital cranial nerve
    b. efferent cranial nerve
    c. radial cranial nerve
    d. seventh cranial nerve
    ____

51. The nerve and branches that supply the thumb side of the arm and back of the hand is the:
    a. buccal nerve
    b. radial nerve
    c. skeletal nerve
    d. posterior nerve ____

52. The anterior tibial nerve extends to the front of the leg, behind the muscles, and is also referred to as:
    a. dorsal nerve
    b. deep peroneal nerve
    c. saphenous nerve
    d. posterior auricular nerve ____

53. The system that controls the steady circulation of blood through the body by means of the heart and blood vessels is the:
    a. capillaries system
    b. circulatory system
    c. skeletal system
    d. lymph system ____

54. The system that involves the heart, arteries, capillaries, and veins is the:
    a. muscular system
    b. blood vascular system
    c. digestive system
    d. respiratory system ____

55. A clear yellowish fluid that circulates in the lymphatics of the body and carries waste and impurities away from the cells is:
    a. pericardium
    b. leukocytes
    c. lymph
    d. blood ____

56. The upper, thin-walled chambers of the heart are the:
    a. left and right pulses
    b. left and right atria
    c. left and right arteries
    d. left and right valves ____

57. The blood circulatory system that sends blood from the heart to the lungs to be purified is the:
    a. ventricle circulation
    b. pulmonary circulation
    c. carotid system
    d. lymphatic drainage system ____

58. Tubelike structures that include arteries, capillaries, and veins are:
    a. heart vessels
    b. valve vessels
    c. blood vessels
    d. platelet vessels ____

59. A thin-walled blood vessel that is less elastic than an artery is a:
    a. vein
    b. vulna
    c. leukocyte
    d. platelet ____

60. The largest artery in the human body is the:
    a. ventricle
    b. capillary
    c. aorta
    d. atrium ____

61. White blood cells perform the important function of destroying:
    a. nonpathogenic organisms
    b. disease-causing microorganisms
    c. internal and external movements
    d. carbon dioxide microorganisms ____

62. The artery that supplies blood to the anterior (front) part of the scalp, ear, face, neck, and side of the head is the:
    a. lymph common artery
    b. mandible cardiac artery
    c. external carotid artery
    d. internal carotid artery ____

63. The main blood supply of the arms and hands are the:
    a. facial and superficial arteries
    b. ulnar and radial arteries
    c. radial and posterior arteries
    d. ulnar and external jugular arteries ____

64. Which of the following is NOT an artery that supplies blood to the lower leg or foot?
    a. popliteal artery
    b. anterior tibial artery
    c. radial artery
    d. posterior tibial artery ____

65. Endocrine glands release a secretion called:
    a. platelets
    b. hormones
    c. enzymes
    d. perspiration ____

66. The integumentary system is made up of the skin and accessory organs such as:
    a. oil and sweat glands, sensory receptors, hair, and nails
    b. diaphragm glands, secondary receptors, and nails
    c. involuntary glands, hair, and hands
    d. cardiac glands, voluntary glands, and nails ____

CHAPTER 7—SKIN STRUCTURE AND GROWTH

1. The medical branch of science that deals with the study of skin, its functions, diseases, and treatment is:
   a. histology
   b. dermatology
   c. elasticity
   d. dermis ____

2. The largest living organ of the body is the:
   a. lungs
   b. heart
   c. skin
   d. neck ____

3. Healthy skin is slightly moist, soft, and flexible with a texture that is:
   a. soft and large pores
   b. smooth and fine-grained
   c. smooth and nonacidic
   d. rough and acidic ____

4. Continued pressure on any part of the skin can cause it to thicken and develop a:
   a. callus
   b. infection
   c. rash
   d. psoriasis ____

5. Appendages of the skin include hair, nails, and:
   a. oil and dirt glands
   b. sweat and keratin glands
   c. sweat and oil glands
   d. oil and pore glands ____

6. The skin structure is generally thinnest on the:
   a. nose
   b. hands
   c. eyebrows
   d. eyelids ____

7. The skin on the scalp has larger and deeper:
   a. nerve endings
   b. hair follicles
   c. keratin layers
   d. blood vessels ____

8. The outermost layer of the skin is also called the:
   a. epidermis layer
   b. dermal layer
   c. thinnest layer
   d. second layer ____

9. The epidermis layer of the skin does not contain:
   a. nerve endings
   b. sweat glands
   c. blood vessels
   d. sensory nerves ____

10. The stratum germinativum is the deepest layer of the epidermis and is responsible for:
    a. growth of the epidermis
    b. strength of the epidermis
    c. nerve endings in the epidermis
    d. sweat and oil glands ____

11. The dark special cells that protect sensitive cells and provide color to the skin are:
    a. reticular
    b. melanocytes
    c. dermis
    d. keratin ____

12. The granular layer of the skin is also called the:
    a. stratum granulosum layer
    b. stratus melanocytes layer
    c. protective layer
    d. adipose tissue layer ____

13. The outermost layer of the epidermis is the:
    a. fiber protein
    b. stratum corneum
    c. lipids layer
    d. second layer ____

14. A fiber protein that is the principal component of hair and nails is:
    a. keratin
    b. melanln
    c. sebum
    d. subcutis ____

15. The deepest layer of the epidermis is the:
    a. horny layer
    b. stratum germinativum
    c. stratum papillae
    d. clear layer ____

16. The clear, transparent layer under the skin surface is the:
    a. subcutaneous tissue
    b. stratum corneum
    c. stratum lucidum
    d. nerve cells ____

17. Cells that are almost dead and pushed to the surface to replace cells are shed from the:
    a. follicles
    b. stratum lucidum layer
    c. fatty skin layer
    d. stratum granulosum layer ____

18. The underlying or inner layer of the skin is the:
    a. dermis layer
    b. epidermis layer
    c. keratin layer
    d. basal layer ____

19. The outermost layer, directly beneath the epidermis, is the:
    a. clear layer
    b. dermal layer
    c. papillary layer
    d. elastin layer ____

20. The deepest layer of the dermis that supplies the skin with oxygen and nutrients and contains sweat and oil glands is the:
    a. regular layer
    b. reticular layer
    c. subcutis layer
    d. highly sensitive layer ____

21. Tissue that gives smoothness and contour to the body and provides a protective cushion is:
    a. subcutaneous tissue
    b. sweat pores
    c. epidermis
    d. basal cell layer ____

22. The clear fluid that removes toxins and cellular waste and has immune functions is:
    a. blood
    b. nerves
    c. corpuscles
    d. lymph ____

23. Motor nerve fibers attached to the hair follicle that can cause goose bumps are the:
    a. arrector pili muscle
    b. body temperature
    c. sebum
    d. melanin ____

24. Nerves that regulate the secretion of perspiration and sebum are:
    a. sweat pores
    b. melanocytes
    c. secretory nerve fibers
    d. tactile corpuscles ____

25. Basic sensations such as touch, pain, heat, cold, and pressure are registered by:
    a. nerve fundus
    b. nerve endings
    c. light
    d. fear ____

26. The amount and type of pigment produced by an individual is determined by:
    a. sun
    b. blood
    c. genes
    d. age ____

27. Two types of melanin produced by the body are:
    a. brown and basal melanin
    b. keratin and elastin
    c. light and red melanin
    d. pheomelanin and eumelanin ____

28. Skin gets its strength, form, and flexibility from flexible fibers found within the:
    a. dermis layer
    b. epidermis layer
    c. true skin
    d. scarf skin ____

29. The fibrous protein that gives skin its form and strength is:
    a. granular
    b. melanin
    c. elastin
    d. collagen ____

30. A fiber that gives skin its flexibility and elasticity is:
    a. elastin
    b. eumelanin
    c. melanin
    d. fibers ____

31. The sudoriferous glands help the body regulate:
    a. dryness
    b. emotions
    c. temperature
    d. blood ____

32. A tubelike duct that ends at the skin surface to form the sweat pore is the:
    a. arrector pili
    b. secretory coil
    c. follicle
    d. papilla ____

33. The sebaceous or oil glands are connected to the:
    a. hair follicle
    b. adipose tissue
    c. nerve endings
    d. blood and lymph ____

34. The principal functions of the skin are protection, sensation, heat regulation. excretion, and:
    a. flexibility and shape
    b. secretion and absorption
    c. strength and muscle tone
    d. hormone balance and repair ____

35. The best way to support the health of the skin is by eating foods from:
    a. carbohydrates, vitamins, and water
    b. fats, oils, and vitamins
    c. water, dairy, and proteins
    d. fats, carbohydrates, and proteins ____

CHAPTER 8—NAIL STRUCTURE AND GROWTH

1. The hard protective plate found at the ends of fingers and toes are:
   a. nail grooves
   b. natural nails
   c. nail ends
   d. mantles
   ____

2. The area under a healthy nail plate should appear:
   a. bluish
   b. reddish
   c. pinkish
   d. brownish
   ____

3. A main protein that is found in natural nails is:
   a. water
   b. keratin
   c. cuticle
   d. melanin
   ____

4. Nails are an appendage of the skin and are part of what body system?
   a. digestive system
   b. respiratory system
   c. nervous system
   d. integumentary system
   ____

5. A healthy nail is smooth, shiny, and:
   a. dark gray
   b. translucent gray
   c. bluish
   d. translucent
   ____

6. The portion of the living skin on which the nail plate sits is the:
   a. nail bed
   b. cuticle
   c. nail fold
   d. ligament
   ____

7. The nail bed is attached to the nail plate by a thin layer of tissue called the:
   a. natural nail
   b. free edge
   c. bed epithelium
   d. nail groove
   ____

8. Nail cells are formed in what part of the nail structure?
   a. matrix
   b. mantle
   c. cuticle
   d. muscles
   ____

9. The nail plate is guided and helped along during its growth by a thin layer of tissue called:
   a. matrix cells
   b. bed epithelium
   c. nail groove
   d. nail enhancement
   ____

10. The matrix continues to create new cells provided that:
    a. it is conditioned with regular manicures
    b. it receives nutrition and is kept healthy
    c. it is attached to the free edge
    d. it extends beyond the free edge
    ____

11. The visible part of the matrix that extends from underneath the living skin is the:
    a. cuticle
    b. root
    c. lunula
    d. bulb
    ____

12. The most visible and functional part of the nail module is the:
    a. nail plate
    b. free edge
    c. cuticle
    d. lunula
    ____

13. The nail plate is constructed of how many layers of nail cells?
    a. 10
    b. 20
    c. 50
    d. 100
    ____

14. The part of the nail plate that extends over the tip of the finger or toe is the:
    a. free edge
    b. manual edge
    c. nail root
    d. nail groove
    ____

15. The dead, colorless tissue attached to the nail plate is:
    a. groove
    b. matrix
    c. cuticle
    d. eponychium
    ____

16. The living skin at the base of the nail plate covering the matrix area is the:
    a. eponychium
    b. hyponychium
    c. cuticle
    d. free edge
    ____

17. The slightly thickened layer of skin that lies underneath the free edge of the nail plate is the:
    a. hyponychium
    b. cuticle
    c. eponychium
    d. nail fold
    ____

18. Tough bands of fibrous tissues that connect bones are:
    a. arteries
    b. ligaments
    c. tendons
    d. mantle
    ____

19. The slits or furrows on the sides of the nail plate are:
    a. artificial nails
    b. natural nails
    c. nail mantles
    d. nail grooves
    ____

20. The length, width, and curvature of nails are determined by the:
    a. matrix shape
    b. bed epithelium
    c. groove shape
    d. furrow shape
    ____

21. In the normal adult, the average rate of nail growth is about:
    a. 1/16 inch per month
    b. 1/4 inch per month
    c. 1 inch per year
    d. 1/10 inch per month
    ____

22. A healthy natural nail will continue to grow provided there is no damage to the:
    a. cuticle
    b. groove
    c. matrix
    d. edge

    ____

23. Replacement of the natural fingernail usually takes about:
    a. 6 to 12 months
    b. 4 to 6 months
    c. 4 to 8 weeks
    d. 2 to 8 months

    ____

24. What fingernail grows the fastest?
    a. middle finger
    b. thumb
    c. toenails
    d. damaged nails

    ____

25. The nail has a water content between:
    a. 10 and 15 percent
    b. 1 and 5 percent
    c. 20 and 45 percent
    d. 15 and 25 percent

    ____

CHAPTER 9—PROPERTIES OF THE HAIR AND SCALP

1. The scientific study of hair, its diseases, and care is called:
   a. dermatology c. biology
   b. trichology d. cosmetology ____

2. The two parts of a mature hair strand are the hair shaft and:
   a. dermis c. hair root
   b. hair follicle d. hair ends ____

3. The portion of hair that projects above the skin is the:
   a. dermal papilla c. hair root
   b. hair shaft d. follicle ____

4. The follicle, bulb, papilla, arrector pili muscle, and sebaceous glands are main structures of the:
   a. hair shaft c. cortex layers
   b. sudoriferous glands d. hair root ____

5. The tubelike depression or pocket in the skin or scalp that contains the hair root is the:
   a. follicle c. bulb
   b. shaft d. scalp ____

6. Hair follicles are not found on the palms of the hands or the:
   a. forehead area c. soles of the feet
   b. elbow area d. back of the neck ____

7. The follicle extends downward from the epidermis, where it surrounds the:
   a. epidermis layer c. hair root
   b. dermal papilla d. hair shaft ____

8. The lowest area or part of the hair strand is the:
   a. hair bulb c. arrector pili
   b. hair shaft d. sebaceous gland ____

9. A small, cone-shaped area at the base of the hair follicle that fits into the hair bulb is the:
   a. sweat pore c. dermal papilla
   b. hair follicle d. lymph gland ____

10. A tiny, involuntary muscle fiber inserted in the base of the hair follicle is the:
    a. dermal papilla c. lanugo hair
    b. arrector pili d. hair bulb ____

11. The oil glands of the skin connected to the hair follicles are:
    a. sweat glands
    b. dermal papilla
    c. sebaceous glands
    d. hair streams ____

12. An oily substance secreted from the sebaceous glands is:
    a. sweat
    b. medulla
    c. sebum
    d. salt ____

13. The overlapping layer of hair with transparent, scalelike cells is the:
    a. bulb
    b. follicle
    c. cuticle
    d. medulla ____

14. The three main layers of the hair shaft are the cuticle, medulla, and:
    a. cortex
    b. shaft
    c. root
    d. bulb ____

15. Swelling the hair raises the cuticle layer and allows for:
    a. primary defense
    b. penetration
    c. cross sections
    d. growth phase ____

16. For chemicals to penetrate a healthy cuticle hair layer, they must:
    a. expose the mantle layer
    b. stiffen the hair shaft
    c. have an alkaline pH
    d. remove the cuticle layer ____

17. The fibrous protein core of the hair, formed by elongated cells containing melanin pigment, is the:
    a. lower follicle
    b. cortex layer
    c. vellus hair
    d. dermal papilla ____

18. The medulla is the innermost layer of the hair and is composed of:
    a. oval cells
    b. round cells
    c. coarse hair
    d. hair follicles ____

19. Hair is composed of a protein that grows from cells originating within the:
    a. hair shaft
    b. hair follicle
    c. amino acids
    d. main elements ____

20. The process whereby living cells mature and begin their journey up the hair shaft is:
    a. simplicity
    b. scalp
    c. keratinization
    d. medulla ____

21. The five main elements that make up the chemical composition of human hair are carbon, oxygen, hydrogen, and:
    a. protein and amino
    b. cells and keratin
    c. elements and protein
    d. nitrogen and sulfur ____

22. The chemical bonds that hold together the amino acid molecules are:
    a. convex bonds
    b. peptide bonds
    c. hydrogen drops
    d. protein cells ____

23. An end bond is also known as a(n):
    a. molecule bond
    b. chain bond
    c. peptide bond
    d. elastic bond ____

24. When peptide bonds hold together a very long chain of amino acids, it is called a:
    a. polypeptide chain
    b. hydrogen chain
    c. COHNS bond
    d. elasticity chain ____

25. The three types of cross-links that form the bonds between the polypeptide chains are hydrogen bonds, salt bonds, and:
    a. disulfide bonds
    b. water bonds
    c. nitrogen bonds
    d. elastic bonds ____

26. A weak type of physical side bond that is easily broken by water or heat is a(n):
    a. amino acid
    b. peptide chain
    c. single bond
    d. hydrogen bond ____

27. A salt bond is easily broken with the use of:
    a. several acidic solutions
    b. conditioning treatments
    c. strong alkaline or acidic solutions
    d. thermal styling techniques ____

28. Bonds that must be chemically separated are:
    a. disulfide bonds
    b. sulfur bonds
    c. cross links
    d. porosity ____

29. Hydrogen chemical hair relaxers break disulfide bonds and during rinsing convert them to:
    a. COHNS bonds
    b. protein bonds
    c. sebum bonds
    d. lanthionine bonds ____

30. The natural hair pigment found in the cortex layer of the hair is:
    a. melanin
    b. tissue
    c. protein
    d. brown ____

31. Two different types of melanin are eumelanin and:
    a. phosphorus
    b. pheomelanin
    c. keratin
    d. sulfur ____

32. Natural wave patterns are the result of:
    a. trichoptilosis
    b. health
    c. structure
    d. genetics ____

33. Asians tend to have:
    a. extremely straight hair
    b. extremely curly hair
    c. straight to wavy hair
    d. wavy to curly hair ____

34. Extremely curly hair grows:
    a. in long twisted spirals
    b. in short curves
    c. in a very regular pattern
    d. with very thick texture ____

35. To help minimize tangles in extremely curly hair when washing, you should use:
    a. a drying shampoo
    b. strong scalp manipulations
    c. a detangling rinse
    d. regular soap instead of shampoo ____

36. Extremely curly hair may often break or knot easily due to:
    a. humidity
    b. density
    c. high elasticity
    d. low elasticity ____

37. Four important factors to consider in hair analysis are texture and porosity:
    a. elasticity and density
    b. dryness and length
    c. oiliness and length
    d. oiliness and color ____

38. The thickness or diameter of the individual hair strand is the:
    a. hair strand
    b. hair porosity
    c. hair texture
    d. hair elasticity ____

39. Hair texture is classified as:
    a. coarse, medium, or fine
    b. coarse, straight, or curly
    c. large or small diameter
    d. long, medium, or short ____

40. The measurement of individual hair strands on one square inch of the scalp is:
    a. hair density
    b. hair structure
    c. hair length
    d. hair porosity ____

41. The ability of the hair to absorb water or oil is:
    a. resistance
    b. porosity
    c. elasticity
    d. texture ____

42. Chemical services performed on hair with low porosity require:
    a. neutral solutions
    b. more acidic solutions
    c. more alkaline solutions
    d. water solutions ____

43. Hair with high porosity is often the result of:
    a. overprocessing
    b. conditioning
    c. too many shampoos
    d. hair texture ____

44. The ability of the hair to stretch and return without breaking is:
    a. elasticity
    b. bounce
    c. porosity
    d. melanin ____

45. Wet hair with normal elasticity will stretch up to:
    a. 25 percent
    b. 40 percent
    c. 50 percent
    d. 70 percent ____

46. When shaping and styling hair, consider the hair's:
    a. length and color
    b. natural growth patterns
    c. natural shine and condition
    d. texture and color ____

47. Dry hair and scalp can be caused by:
    a. inactive sebaceous glands
    b. alkaline water
    c. dry shampoos
    d. flaky scalp ____

48. Oily scalp and hair can be treated by properly shampooing with:
    a. alkaline shampoo
    b. normalizing shampoo
    c. color shampoo
    d. warm water ____

49. Hair that is not pigmented and almost never has a medulla is:
    a. oily
    b. pigmented
    c. dark
    d. vellus ____

50. Long, soft hair found on the scalp, legs, arms, and bodies of males and females is:
    a. average
    b. scabies
    c. terminal
    d. vellum ____

51. The phases of hair growth are anagen, catagen, and:
    a. telogen
    b. melanin
    c. repeated
    d. carbuncle ____

52. The growth phase where new hair is produced is:
    a. transition
    b. telogen
    c. anagen
    d. regular ____

53. The average growth of healthy scalp hair is:
    a. one half inch per week
    b. one half inch per year
    c. three quarters of an inch per month
    d. one inch per month ____

54. The final or resting phase in the hair growth cycle is:
    a. broken stage
    b. telogen stage
    c. anagen stage
    d. hypertrichosis stage ____

55. In general, the cross sections of curly hair can be:
    a. oval
    b. triangular
    c. even
    d. square ____

56. The term used to identify abnormal hair loss is:
    a. androgenic
    b. alopecia
    c. areata
    d. genetic ____

57. The sudden falling out of hair in round patches or baldness in spots is called:
    a. terminal hair
    b. hypertrichosis
    c. alopecia areata
    d. alopecia androgenic ____

58. Two products approved by the FDA to stimulate hair growth and allowed for sale in the United States are:
    a. minoxidil and finasteride
    b. tinea and medication
    c. conditioning and rogaine
    d. finasteride and antiseptics ____

59. The technical term used to describe gray hair is:
    a. albinos
    b. acquired
    c. alopecia
    d. canities ____

60. A variety of canities, characterized by alternating bands of gray and pigmented hair, is:
    a. ringed hair
    b. alopecia areata
    c. hypertrichosis
    d. trichoptilosis ____

61. A condition of abnormal hair growth on areas of the body is:
    a. trichorrhexis
    b. hyperactive
    c. hypertrichosis
    d. electrolysis ____

62. Trichorrhexis nodosa is characterized by brittleness of the hair and the formation of:
    a. swellings along the hair shaft
    b. split ends along the hair shaft
    c. lubricated dry ends
    d. alternating bands of color ____

63. The technical term used to describe beaded hair is:
    a. monilethrix
    b. monoglycerine
    c. finasteride
    d. fragile ____

64. The medical term for dandruff is:
    a. canities
    b. pityriasis
    c. alopecia
    d. simplex ____

65. The medical term used to describe a fungal organism characterized by itching, scales, and painful circular lesions is:
    a. scapular
    b. seborrheic
    c. tinea
    d. alopecia ____

66. The type of fungal infection characterized by red papules at the opening of the hair follicles is:
    a. tinea capitis
    b. pediculosis
    c. steatoides
    d. pityriasis ____

67. A highly contagious skin disease caused by a mite parasite is:
    a. scabies
    b. capitis
    c. infestation
    d. furuncles ____

68. An acute localized bacterial infection of the hair follicle that produces constant pain is:
    a. a furuncle
    b. scabies
    c. pediculosis
    d. carbuncle ____

69. An inflammation of the subcutaneous tissue caused by staphylococci is:
    a. a carbuncle
    b. pediculosis
    c. anagen
    d. alopecia ____

70. The spread of diseases can be prevented by practicing approved:
    a. healthy diet and exercise
    b. sanitation and disinfection procedures
    c. various options
    d. hair analysis procedures ____

CHAPTER 10—BASICS OF CHEMISTRY

1. The science that deals with the composition, structures, and properties of matter and how matter changes under different conditions is known as:
   a. compounds
   b. chemistry
   c. electricity
   d. structural changes ____

2. The study of substances that contain carbon is referred to as:
   a. inorganic chemistry
   b. chemical composition
   c. organic chemistry
   d. natural products ____

3. Products manufactured from natural gas, oil, or plant or animal remains are considered to be:
   a. organic
   b. natural
   c. inorganic
   d. matter ____

4. Metals, minerals, water, and air are examples of :
   a. natural substances
   b. inorganic substances
   c. compounds
   d. proteins ____

5. Inorganic chemistry is the science that deals with compounds lacking:
   a. lead
   b. silver
   c. carbon
   d. water ____

6. Any substance that occupies space and has mass can be considered to be:
   a. simple
   b. matter
   c. energy
   d. inorganic ____

7. A basic substance that cannot be broken down into simpler substances without loss of identity is called:
   a. a compound
   b. water
   c. a molecule
   d. an element ____

8. Substances that cannot be divided into simpler substances by ordinary chemical means are:
   a. atoms
   b. inorganic
   c. chemical
   d. atomic ____

9. The smallest particle of an element is a(n):
   a. hydrogen
   b. atom
   c. axle
   d. acid ____

10. Chemically joining two or more atoms forms a(n):
    a. acid
    b. molecule
    c. mixture
    d. solvent ____

11. Chemical combinations of two or more atoms of different elements form:
    a. a mixture
    b. silicone
    c. oxygen
    d. a compound ____

12. Normal matter exists in three different physical states, which are solid, gas, and:
    a. liquid
    b. organic
    c. air
    d. solute ____

13. Characteristics that do not involve chemically changing a substance are:
    a. unique properties
    b. mechanical properties
    c. physical properties
    d. distinct characteristics ____

14. A change in a substance's chemical composition is a:
    a. natural change
    b. chemical change
    c. chemical mixture
    d. chemical synthesis ____

15. Matter that is not mixed with substances of different chemical compositions is a:
    a. pure substance
    b. physical substance
    c. chemical reaction
    d. compatible substance ____

16. Physical mixtures containing two or more different substances are:
    a. suspensions, chemicals, and matter
    b. solutions, suspensions, and emulsions
    c. compounds, physical matter, and water
    d. minerals, compounds, and emulsions ____

17. A blended mixture of two or more liquids or a solid dissolved in a liquid is a(n):
    a. solution
    b. emulsion
    c. compound
    d. alkaline ____

18. A substance that dissolves another substance with no change in chemical composition is a:
    a. solute
    b. mineral
    c. solvent
    d. mixture ____

19. Miscible liquids are liquids that can be:
    a. mixed without shaking
    b. mixed into stable solutions
    c. transformed into a suspension
    d. combined without a solvent ____

20. Liquids that are not capable of being mixed into stable solutions are:
    a. solutes
    b. solvents
    c. inverted
    d. immiscible ____

21. A product that does not separate when standing and contains particles is considered to be:
    a. organic
    b. a solvent
    c. a solution
    d. a mixture ____

22. Solutions that contain undissolved particles that are visible to the naked eye are known as:
    a. suspensions
    b. mixtures
    c. solutes
    d. molecules ____

23. A mixture of two or more immiscible substances united with the aid of a binder is known as a(n):
    a. suspension
    b. emulsion
    c. mixture
    d. solution ____

24. A substance that acts as a bridge to allow oil and water to mix or emulsify is a(n):
    a. active agent
    b. surfactant
    c. alkaline
    d. deionization ____

25. The water-loving head of a surfactant molecule is:
    a. hydrogen
    b. lipophilic
    c. hydrophilic
    d. neutral ____

26. Ammonium hydroxide and ammonium thioglycolate are examples of products used to:
    a. raise the pH of hair
    b. neutralize the pH of hair
    c. compose hydrogen bonds
    d. neutralize the hair ____

27. An atom or molecule that carries an electric charge is an:
    a. arc
    b. acid
    c. ion
    d. alkaline ____

28. Acids owe their chemical reactivity to the:
    a. chemical compounds
    b. hydrogen ion
    c. hydrogen peroxide
    d. neutralization solute ____

29. Chemical reactions that produce heat are called:
    a. external
    b. emulsions
    c. redox
    d. exothermic ____

30. The chemical reaction that combines an element or compound with oxygen to produce an oxide is:
    a. suspension
    b. reduction
    c. neutralization
    d. oxidation ____

31. The rapid oxidation of any substance accompanied by heat or light is:
    a. oxygen
    b. combustion
    c. protons
    d. electricity ____

32. When oxygen is subtracted from a substance, the chemical reaction is called:
    a. release
    b. reduction
    c. oxidized
    d. redox ____

33. A substance that has a pH above 7.0 is considered to be a(n):
    a. neutral solution
    b. acid solution
    c. alkali solution
    d. reducing solution ____

34. A sweet, colorless, oily substance used as a moisturizing ingredient in cosmetic products is:
    a. glycerin
    b. moisturizing
    c. ointment
    d. compound ____

35. The chemical reaction in which the oxidizing agent is reduced and the reducing agent is oxidized is:
    a. redox
    b. reducing
    c. neutral
    d. solute ____

CHAPTER 11—BASICS OF ELECTRICITY

1. Electricity is described as a form of:
   a. energy
   b. movement
   c. negativity
   d. shortness
   ____

2. The flow of electricity along a conductor is called a(n):
   a. electric charge
   b. electric current
   c. swirl
   d. spark
   ____

3. Metals used in electric wiring and motors are materials that are considered good electricity:
   a. current
   b. conductors
   c. wattage
   d. ohms
   ____

4. Electric wires are usually covered with a rubber substance that is used as an insulator or:
   a. nonconductor
   b. mechanical
   c. current
   d. voltage
   ____

5. The path of electricity from the generating source through conductors and back to the original source is called a(n):
   a. electric charge
   b. alternating charge
   c. insulator
   d. complete circuit
   ____

6. Electric current that is constant, even-flowing and travels in one direction is:
   a. direct current
   b. direct volt
   c. converter
   d. active current
   ____

7. The device that changes direct current to alternating current is a(n):
   a. convex
   b. converter
   c. voltage
   d. ohm
   ____

8. A rapid and interrupted current that flows in one direction then in the opposite direction is:
   a. rectifier current
   b. alternating current
   c. active current
   d. direct current
   ____

9. The unit that measures the pressure or force that pushes the flow of electrons through a conductor is a(n):
   a. amp
   b. rectifier
   c. apparatus
   d. volt
   ____

10. The unit that measures the amount of electric current is a(n):
    a. battery
    b. volt
    c. ampere
    d. charger
    ____

11. The current that is used for facial and scalp treatments is measured in:
    a. milliamperes
    b. direct current
    c. wattage
    d. voltage
    ____

12. The unit that measures how much electric energy is being used in one second is a(n):
    a. ohm
    b. watt
    c. amp
    d. volt
    ____

13. The device that prevents excessive current from passing through a circuit is a(n):
    a. fuse
    b. battery
    c. kilowatt
    d. ampere
    ____

14. A switch that automatically interrupts or shuts off an electric current at the first indication of an overload is a(n):
    a. voltage regulator
    b. ampere current
    c. circuit breaker
    d. battery charger
    ____

15. An important way of promoting electrical safety is the principle of:
    a. grounding
    b. connections
    c. low frequency
    d. visible light
    ____

16. An applicator that is used for directing the electric current from the machine to the client's skin is called a(n):
    a. steamer
    b. anaphoresis
    c. polarity
    d. electrode
    ____

17. The positive electrode of an electrotherapy device is called a(n):
    a. frequency
    b. anode
    c. vaporizer
    d. accelerating
    ____

18. The negative electrode of an electrotherapy device is called a(n):
    a. cathode
    b. electron
    c. carbon
    d. therapeutic
    ____

19. The most commonly used modality that is a constant and direct current is:
    a. indirect current
    b. active current
    c. galvanic current
    d. Tesla current
    ____

20. The process of introducing water-soluble products into the skin with the use of electric current is called:
    a. chemical reaction
    b. inactive electrodes
    c. iontophoresis
    d. electrodes
    ____

21. A process that forces liquids into the tissues from the negative toward the positive pole is called:
    a. anaphoresis
    b. desincrustation
    c. iontophoresis
    d. therapeutic light

    ____

22. A thermal or heat-producing current with a high rate of oscillation that is used for scalp and facial treatments is:
    a. Tesla current
    b. direct current
    c. alternating current
    d. infrared current

    ____

23. Visible light, the part of the electromagnetic radiation spectrum that we can see, makes up what percentage of natural sunlight?
    a. 35 percent
    b. 25 percent
    c. 60 percent
    d. 50 percent

    ____

24. The long wavelengths that penetrate the deepest and produce the most heat are:
    a. infrared rays
    b. blue rays
    c. ultraviolet rays
    d. natural rays

    ____

25. To avoid damage to the eyes of a client or practitioner when using light therapy treatments, the eyes should be protected with saturated cotton pads or:
    a. safety goggles
    b. sunscreen
    c. plastic cap
    d. towels

    ____

CHAPTER 12—PRINCIPLES OF HAIR DESIGN

1. The foundation for all artistic applications is:
   a. space
   b. design
   c. design wave patterns
   d. design of parallel lines ____

2. The design process begins by analyzing the entire person and using the design elements and principles to:
   a. enhance positive features
   b. maximize negative features
   c. develop contrasting lines
   d. create transitional lines ____

3. In the hair design process, when deciding to take calculated risks, it is important to have a strong foundation in:
   a. confidence and balance
   b. fashion design
   c. techniques and skills
   d. form and space ____

4. In the principles of design, line defines:
   a. form and space
   b. less volume
   c. texture and form
   d. form and elements ____

5. Lines that extend in the same direction and maintain a constant distance apart are:
   a. design lines
   b. extended lines
   c. horizontal lines
   d. vertical lines ____

6. Lines positioned between horizontal and vertical, used to emphasize or minimize facial features, are:
   a. curved lines
   b. movement lines
   c. design lines
   d. diagonal lines ____

7. An example of a hairstyle created using a single line is a:
   a. contrasting style
   b. curved-line style
   c. monotone style
   d. one-length style ____

8. Curved lines that are used to blend and soften horizontal or vertical lines are:
   a. transitional lines
   b. styling lines
   c. contrasting lines
   d. parallel lines ____

9. The three-dimensional mass or general outline of a hairstyle is referred to as its:
   a. wave
   b. form
   c. weight
   d. line ____

10. In hairstyling, the area that surrounds the form is the:
    a. space
    b. line
    c. volume
    d. texture ____

11. Natural wave patterns are described as straight, wavy, curly, and:
    a. three-dimensional
    b. very straight
    c. combination
    d. extremely curly
    ____

12. In hair design, with every movement, the relationship of form and what other design element change?
    a. space
    b. volume
    c. texture
    d. mass
    ____

13. Hair texture changes can be created or changed temporarily with styling tools and permanently with:
    a. thermal styling
    b. chemicals
    c. zigzag partings
    d. flat irons
    ____

14. Smooth wave patterns accent the face and can be used to narrow:
    a. a square jaw
    b. rectangular features
    c. a square chin
    d. a round head shape
    ____

15. Illusions of dimension or depth are created when lighter and warmer colors are alternated with colors that are:
    a. darker and cooler
    b. smaller and closer
    c. larger and darker
    d. smaller and cooler
    ____

16. For a client with gold skin tones, a flattering hair color tone would be:
    a. warm
    b. cool
    c. contrasting
    d. toned
    ____

17. In the principles of art and design, the comparative relationship of one thing to another is called:
    a. space
    b. volume
    c. proportion
    d. harmony
    ____

18. In designing for clients with large or broad shoulders, the stylist would create styles with:
    a. volume
    b. length
    c. classic
    d. shape
    ____

19. Balance is described as creating equal or appropriate proportions to create:
    a. width
    b. symmetry
    c. structure
    d. space
    ____

20. In designing, when the two sides are the same distance from the center, have the same length and volume, the balance is considered to be:
    a. symmetrical
    b. even
    c. asymmetrical
    d. similar ____

21. In designing, when opposite sides have different lengths or different volume and appear to have equal visual weight, it is referred to as:
    a. rhythm balance
    b. positioned evenly
    c. symmetrical balance
    d. asymmetrical balance ____

22. A recurrent pattern of movement in design is referred to as:
    a. rhythm
    b. diagonal
    c. shapings
    d. balance ____

23. The area of a design where the eye is drawn to first before traveling to the rest of the design is called the:
    a. balance
    b. axis
    c. emphasis
    d. diagonal ____

24. The most important art principle that holds a design together is:
    a. harmony
    b. balance
    c. volume
    d. emphasis ____

25. The facial type that is about one and a half times longer than its width across the brow is the:
    a. oval face
    b. oblong face
    c. facial contour
    d. diamond face ____

26. To offset or round out the features of a square facial shape, the aim would be to:
    a. create the illusion of width in the forehead
    b. add volume to top and closeness at the sides
    c. elongate the shape of the face
    d. create volume between the temples and jaw ____

27. The facial shape with a narrow forehead and wide jaw and chin line is considered to be:
    a. square
    b. oval
    c. triangular
    d. diamond ____

28. The face profile with a receding forehead and chin is generally referred to as:
    a. concave
    b. circular
    c. straight
    d. convex ____

29. To give the illusion of proportional eyes to a client with wide-set eyes, the hair should be:
    a. slightly darker at the sides than top
    b. styled using a middle part
    c. straight lines at the jawbone
    d. full and below jaw ____

30. The triangular section that begins at the apex or high point of the head and ends at the front corners is called the:
    a. crown area
    b. bang area
    c. line area
    d. convex area ____

CHAPTER 13—SHAMPOOING, RINSING, AND CONDITIONING

1. The shampoo provides a good opportunity for the stylist to analyze the client's:
   a. hair and scalp conditions
   b. hair and facial features
   c. hair and makeup
   d. scalp and makeup ____

2. A client with an infectious disease should be referred to a:
   a. stylist
   b. treatment
   c. physician
   d. client ____

3. The primary purpose of a shampoo is to:
   a. recommend additional services
   b. cleanse the hair and scalp
   c. recommend products
   d. analyze scalp condition ____

4. In the shampoo selection process, understanding the pH scale helps the stylist:
   a. affect the look of a bad haircut for the client
   b. retail products to the client
   c. select the proper shampoo for the client
   d. determine an appropriate style for the client ____

5. An abundant and important element classified as a universal solvent is:
   a. salt
   b. soap
   c. detergent
   d. water ____

6. An alkaline shampoo with a high pH can leave the hair dry, brittle, and more porous and cause fading in:
   a. conditioning rinses
   b. color-treated hair
   c. relaxed hair
   d. virgin hair ____

7. Freshwater from lakes and streams is purified by the processes of sedimentation and:
   a. porous substance
   b. minerals
   c. filtration
   d. organic ____

8. Small amounts of chlorine can be added to water to:
   a. kill bacteria
   b. add minerals
   c. soften water
   d. add dimension ____

9. Water that contains certain minerals that lessen the ability of shampoo to lather readily is:
   a. rain water
   b. soft water
   c. hard water
   d. distilled water ____

10. In listing the ingredients of a product, the percentage of each ingredient is listed in:
    a. descending order
    b. regular order
    c. order of weight
    d. ascending order ____

11. The second ingredient that most shampoos have in common is the primary surfactant or:
    a. color additive
    b. preservative
    c. conditioning agent
    d. base detergent ____

12. The water-attracting end of a surfactant molecule is the:
    a. element
    b. hydrophilic
    c. agent
    d. hydroxide ____

13. An acid-balanced shampoo has a pH in the range of:
    a. 4.0 to 6.0
    b. 4.5 to 5.5
    c. 4.0 to 6.0
    d. 5.0 to 5.5 ____

14. Shampoos that are recommended for use on color-treated or lightened hair are:
    a. alkaline-balanced
    b. detergent based
    c. surfactant free
    d. acid-balanced ____

15. Shampoos with an acidic ingredient used to remove product buildup on hair are:
    a. clarifying shampoos
    b. treatment shampoos
    c. rinsing shampoos
    d. dandruff shampoos ____

16. Shampoos used for oily hair and scalp that remove excess oiliness and keep the hair from drying out are:
    a. dry shampoos
    b. conditioning shampoos
    c. balancing shampoos
    d. color-enhancing shampoos ____

17. Shampoos used to brighten or eliminate unwanted gold or brassiness are:
    a. color-enhancing shampoos
    b. conditioning shampoos
    c. neutralizing shampoos
    d. conditioning shampoos ____

18. Substances that absorb moisture or promote the retention of moisture are:
    a. texturizers
    b. melanins
    c. shampoos
    d. humectants ____

19. A product that slightly increases the diameter of the hair with a coating action, adding body to the hair, is:
    a. protein conditioner
    b. balancing treatment
    c. color enhancer
    d. instant conditioner ____

20. A product that is used after a scalp treatment and before styling to remove oil accumulation is a:
    a. scalp neutralizer
    b. scalp astringent lotion
    c. balancing treatment
    d. conditioning treatment ____

21. Brushing of the hair should never be done prior to:
    a. chemical services
    b. shampoo services
    c. styling services
    d. conditioning services ____

22. The most highly recommended hairbrushes are those made from:
    a. nylon bristles
    b. thermal bristles
    c. natural bristles
    d. smooth bristles ____

23. To avoid physical problems during the shampoo, the correct posture is to:
    a. keep shoulders down and feet together
    b. stand as close as possible to the client
    c. keep shoulders back, abdomen in
    d. stand behind the client ____

24. After shampooing chemically treated hair, gently remove tangles beginning:
    a. at the front hairline and working down to the nape area
    b. at the nape and working up to the frontal area
    c. at the nape area and working sideways
    d. at the frontal area and work toward the ears ____

25. As a safety feature for the client, during a shampoo, the water temperature should be monitored by the stylist by:
    a. adjusting the volume and temperature of the water from hot to cold
    b. keeping one finger over the edge of the spray nozzle in contact with the water
    c. not adjusting the volume and the temperature of the water
    d. keeping the water pressure as high as possible for contact with one finger ____

26. Firm pressure and/or heavy scalp massage should not be administered during the shampoo procedure if the client is to receive a:
    a. client consultation
    b. leave-in conditioner
    c. conditioner pack
    d. chemical service ____

27. After a shampoo, it is not recommended to apply a conditioner:
    a. to the base of the hair, near the scalp
    b. midsection and ends of the hair shaft
    c. to the ends of hair shaft
    d. with massage movements ____

28. A shampoo that is performed when the client's health does not allow for a wet shampoo is a:
    a. dry shampoo procedure
    b. conditioning shampoo procedure
    c. weekly shampoo procedure
    d. medicated shampoo procedure ____

29. A stylist should recommend hair or scalp treatments only after performing a:
    a. scalp consultation
    b. professional service
    c. hair and scalp analysis
    d. shampoo procedure ____

30. A scalp treatment used when there is a deficiency of natural oil on the hair or scalp should contain:
    a. moisturizers and emollient ingredients
    b. sulfonated oil base products
    c. strong soap preparations
    d. mineral and greasy preparations ____

31. High-frequency current should never be used when the hair is treated with tonics that contain:
    a. dirt
    b. alcohol
    c. oils
    d. moisture ____

32. The overactive glands that produce excessive oiliness are the:
    a. hair follicles
    b. arrector pili glands
    c. sebaceous glands
    d. sweat glands ____

33. Dandruff is the result of a fungus called:
    a. malassezia
    b. scabies
    c. pathogenic
    d. tinea ____

34. Alcohol-based antidandruff lotions and tonics should not be used in conjunction with:
    a. thermal styling
    b. scalp massage
    c. filtration
    d. infrared lamps ____

35. When working a shampoo into a lather, the stylist should use:
    a. portion of nails
    b. cushions of fingertips
    c. long fingernails
    d. the wrists ____

CHAPTER 14—HAIRCUTTING

1. A good haircut begins with an understanding of the:
   a. body form
   b. head form
   c. body posture
   d. facial expression ____

2. The areas of the head where the surface of the head changes are:
   a. subsections
   b. starting points
   c. reference points
   d. apex points ____

3. In the haircutting procedure, reference points are used to establish:
   a. head shape
   b. design lines
   c. blunt cutting
   d. foundation lines ____

4. The widest part of the head, also known as the crest area, is the:
   a. apex area
   b. irregular area
   c. occipital area
   d. parietal ridge ____

5. The bone that protrudes at the base of the skull is the:
   a. occipital bone
   b. parietal bone
   c. frontal bone
   d. crest bone ____

6. The highest point at the top of the head is the:
   a. crown
   b. apex
   c. parietal
   d. occipital ____

7. The reference point that signals a change in head shape from flat to round or vice versa is the:
   a. crown area
   b. occipital corner
   c. four corners
   d. parietal ridge ____

8. The area at the back part of the neck below the occipital bone is the:
   a. guide area
   b. flat area
   c. ends area
   d. nape area ____

9. The triangle section that begins at the apex and ends at the front corners is the:
   a. fringe area
   b. front area
   c. corner area
   d. nape area ____

10. A thin continuous mark that is used throughout a haircut is called a(n):
    a. section
    b. corner
    c. angle
    d. line ____

11. The space between two lines or surfaces that intersect at a given point is a(n):
    a. corner
    b. angle
    c. bang
    d. line
    ____

12. The straight lines used to build weight or create a one-length or low-elevation haircut are:
    a. parallel lines
    b. horizontal lines
    c. weight lines
    d. diagonal lines
    ____

13. The straight lines used to remove weight or create graduated layers are:
    a. cutting lines
    b. diagonal lines
    c. vertical lines
    d. horizontal lines
    ____

14. The haircutting technique using diagonal lines to create fullness and blend long layers into short layers is:
    a. beveling
    b. weight
    c. diagonal
    d. fullness
    ____

15. For control during haircutting, the hair is divided into uniform working areas called:
    a. foundations
    b. uneven
    c. parts
    d. sections
    ____

16. The angle or degree at which a subsection of hair is held while cutting is:
    a. subsection
    b. elevation
    c. parting
    d. separating
    ____

17. Elevating the hair at 90 degrees or higher during a haircut results in the removal of:
    a. length and curl
    b. less graduation
    c. weight, or layering the hair
    d. bulk and length
    ____

18. The angle at which the fingers are held when performing a haircut is the:
    a. end shape
    b. blunt cut
    c. cutting line
    d. perimeter line
    ____

19. The first section cut when creating a shape is the:
    a. occipital line
    b. internal part
    c. guideline
    d. basic line
    ____

20. The outer line of a haircut is referred to as the:
    a. traveling guide
    b. stationary guide
    c. interior
    d. perimeter
    ____

21. The guideline used when creating layers or a graduated cut is a:
    a. traveling guideline
    b. outer guideline
    c. stationary guideline
    d. shape guideline

    ____

22. The technique of combing hair away from its natural falling position, rather than straight out from the head toward a guideline, is:
    a. subsectioning
    b. overdirection
    c. traveling guidelines
    d. undercutting

    ____

23. A conversation where the stylist offers professional advice and suggestions to the client is the:
    a. decision process
    b. suggestion process
    c. finished consultation
    d. client consultation

    ____

24. For a client with a long face, the stylist would recommend a style that:
    a. adds volume and height on top
    b. adds fullness on the sides to add width
    c. adds weight to chin and front
    d. adds fullness in length

    ____

25. To compensate for shrinkage associated with curly hair, the stylist should allow for shrinkage of:
    a. 1/4 inch to 1 inch
    b. 1/2 inch to 2 inches
    c. 1/8 inch to 1 inch
    d. 1 inch to 3 inches

    ____

26. The direction that hair grows from the scalp into a natural falling position is the:
    a. outermost perimeter
    b. growth pattern
    c. parallel section
    d. fringe area

    ____

27. The number of individual hair strands on one square inch of scalp is hair:
    a. texture
    b. crown
    c. density
    d. length

    ____

28. The haircutting tool with large teeth set far apart, designed to remove a significant amount of hair, is:
    a. haircutting shears
    b. edger shears
    c. clipper shears
    d. notching shears

    ____

29. A small haircutting tool used to create crisp outlines is a:
    a. feather blade
    b. trimmer
    c. razor
    d. texture shear

    ____

30. The haircutting tool used for close tapers in the scissors-over-comb technique is the:
    a. wide-toothed comb
    b. barber comb
    c. tail comb
    d. styling comb ____

31. The hand that holds the shears, parts the hair, and cuts the hair during the cutting procedure is called the:
    a. holding hand
    b. right hand
    c. dominant hand
    d. extra hand ____

32. The technique where the comb and shears are held closed in the dominant hand at the same time is called:
    a. palming the shears
    b. controlling the shears
    c. opening the shears
    d. holding the comb ____

33. The technique used to free up the dominant cutting hand to cut a subsection is called:
    a. moving the shears
    b. transferring the comb
    c. removing the shears
    d. working the shears ____

34. A haircutting tool used for detailing and texturizing or an entire haircut is the:
    a. shingling
    b. trimmer
    c. straight razor
    d. carving ____

35. The term used to describe the pressure applied to hair when combing or holding a subsection is:
    a. tension
    b. sectioning
    c. elevation
    d. angle ____

36. When cutting straight hair to create a precise design line, use:
    a. no tension
    b. maximum tension
    c. tension ranges
    d. little tension ____

37. When cutting hair, a general rule of thumb is to stand or sit:
    a. directly behind the area you are cutting
    b. directly in front of the area you are cutting
    c. indirectly behind the area you are cutting
    d. to the left of the area you are cutting ____

38. In cutting uniform or increasing layers, the hand position most often used is cutting:
    a. at the fingertips
    b. between the fingers
    c. past the first knuckle
    d. over the fingers ____

39. The technique of cutting below the fingers or inside the knuckles using a horizontal cutting line creates:
    a. cutting uniform or increasing layers
    b. heavier graduated haircut or a one-length bob
    c. shorter layer haircut or a shag effect
    d. high level layered effect or a bi-level cut ____

40. A haircutting technique that maintains control of a subsection with regard to elevations and overdirection is:
    a. cutting over the fingers
    b. cutting with a razor
    c. cutting palm-to-palm
    d. cutting below the fingers ____

41. When cutting below the finger, to prevent cutting the soft and fleshy part of the finger, avoid cutting past:
    a. the second knuckle
    b. the fingertip
    c. the index finger
    d. the thumb ____

42. The visual line in a haircut, where the ends of the hair hang together, is the:
    a. guideline
    b. weight line
    c. graduated line
    d. stationary line ____

43. A haircut achieved using a stationary guide and zero or no elevation and the hair comes to one hanging level is a:
    a. graduated cut
    b. long layers cut
    c. layer cut
    d. blunt cut ____

44. In a graduated haircut, the most common elevation used is:
    a. 0 degrees
    b. 45 degrees
    c. 80 degrees
    d. 30 degrees ____

45. Parting the haircut in the opposite way it was cut to check for precision of line and shape is:
    a. cross-checking
    b. consistent tension
    c. mirror elevation
    d. blunt cutting ____

46. The area of the head that has the most irregular growth patterns is the:
    a. nape
    b. back
    c. crown
    d. sides ____

47. In using the wide teeth of a comb when cutting, comb the section first with the fine teeth and then:
    a. change the position of the comb and comb with fine teeth
    b. switch comb to alternate hand and comb with fine teeth
    c. turn the comb around and comb with the wide teeth
    d. turn the comb on its side and comb with fine teeth ____

48. In general a razor should not be used on curly hair as it will:
    a. strengthen the weight line and cause the hair to frizz
    b. weaken the cuticle and cause the hair to frizz
    c. cause the hair to expand and the medulla to frizz
    d. strengthen the cuticle and cause the hair to flatten ____

49. The term used to describe how hair is moved over the head is:
    a. natural head form
    b. natural distribution
    c. natural fringe
    d. weight line ____

50. When working with a razor, the ends are cut at an angle producing a softer shape with more visible separation or:
    a. blunt effect
    b. short effect
    c. feathered effect
    d. geometric effect ____

51. A method of cutting or thinning hair where the fingers and shears glide along the edge of the hair to remove length is:
    a. angle cutting
    b. razor cutting
    c. slide cutting
    d. blunt cutting ____

52. The scissors-over-comb technique uses the comb to hold the hair in place and allows cutting from:
    a. side to side layers
    b. extremely short to longer lengths
    c. alternating subsections
    d. slightly elevated sides ____

53. The technique of removing excess bulk or cutting for effect without shortening hair length is:
    a. blunt cutting
    b. angle cutting
    c. texturizing
    d. compensating ____

54. Vertical point cutting performed with shears on the ends of hair:
    a. creates no effect
    b. removes gray hair
    c. removes long hair
    d. removes less hair ____

55. When performing the notching technique of texturizing with shears, the tips of the shears should be held:
    a. 5 inches from the ends
    b. 2 inches from the ends
    c. at the ends only
    d. at the midshaft section ____

56. Thinning hair to graduated lengths using a sliding movement with shear blades partially open is:
    a. slithering
    b. notching
    c. point cutting
    d. angle cutting ____

57. The slicing technique removes bulk and adds:
    a. stability through the lengths of the hair
    b. movement through the lengths of the hair
    c. layers and short lengths throughout the hair
    d. density through the lengths of the hair ____

58. When performing the slicing technique on the surface of the haircut, it is best to work on:
    a. long hair
    b. curly hair
    c. dry hair
    d. wet hair ____

59. A version of the slicing technique that creates a visual separation in the hair is:
    a. carving
    b. notching
    c. thinning
    d. pulling ____

60. A tool attached to clippers that cuts the hair to the exact length is:
    a. clippers-over-comb
    b. length guard attachment attachment
    c. taper guard attachment
    d. blended elevation ____

61. With a regular cutting comb, the finer shaped teeth are geared for detailing, and the wider spaced teeth are geared for:
    a. slicing and angle cutting
    b. removing length and detailing
    c. combing and cutting
    d. edging a line ____

62. When using the clipper-over-comb technique, the length is determined by the:
    a. apex of the head
    b. angle of the comb
    c. size of the section
    d. type of clipper used ____

63. Cutting hair at the same length consistently, using a 90-degree elevation, produces a:
    a. uniform layer
    b. blunt cut
    c. one-length bob
    d. slide cut ____

64. In the carving technique, to remove less hair, the scissors should be held:
    a. more open
    b. more closed
    c. more horizontal
    d. more vertical ____

65. Clippers and trimmers should be cleaned and the detachable blade and heel disinfected:
    a. after each use
    b. daily
    c. when needed
    d. weekly ____

CHAPTER 15—HAIRSTYLING

1. To ensure that the client has the knowledge necessary to care for their hair properly between salon visits, it is the responsibility of the professional to:
   a. never explain about proper home care maintenance
   b. educate clients on home hair maintenance and professional products
   c. suggest they purchase consumer products
   d. never suggest the use of professional products ____

2. The first step in the hairstyling process should always be a:
   a. cool water shampoo
   b. draping procedure
   c. client consultation
   d. conditioning treatment ____

3. Shaping and directing the hair into an S formation using a comb, lotion, and the fingers is called:
   a. hairstyling
   b. finger waving
   c. ridge curls
   d. roller setting ____

4. Hair gel that makes the hair pliable, keeps it in place, and is made from karaya gum is:
   a. conditioning gel
   b. diluted gel
   c. waving lotion
   d. hair conditioner ____

5. When creating finger waves with a side part, you should begin on the:
   a. drying side
   b. heavy side
   c. control side
   d. triangle side ____

6. In creating horizontal finger waves, the waves are placed:
   a. up and down the head
   b. on the heavy side of the head
   c. down and parallel
   d. sideways and parallel around the head ____

7. The stationary foundation of a pin curl is the:
   a. base
   b. curl
   c. section
   d. stem ____

8. The part of a pin curl that gives the curl its direction and movement is the:
   a. arc
   b. stem
   c. base
   d. no-stem ____

9. The stem of the pin curl is the part that determines:
   a. placement
   b. curl
   c. width
   d. mobility ____

10. Pin curls that produce tight, firm, long-lasting curls and allow for minimum mobility are:
    a. no-stem pin curl
    b. half-stem pin curl
    c. on-base pin curl
    d. off-base pin curl
    ____

11. Pin curls formed in a shaping should begin at the:
    a. open end
    b. closed side
    c. odd side
    d. shaping side
    ____

12. Smooth waves and uniform curls are produced by:
    a. closed center curls
    b. no-stem curls
    c. open center curls
    d. molded curls
    ____

13. Pin curls formed in the opposite direction of the hands of a clock are:
    a. alternating curls
    b. counterclockwise curls
    c. clockwise curls
    d. ridge curls
    ____

14. Pin curl bases are referred to as rectangular, triangular, square, or:
    a. arc-based
    b. on-base
    c. no-base
    d. closed-base
    ____

15. Triangular base pin curls are used along the front or facial hairline to:
    a. provide volume and height
    b. add wave patterns
    c. provide smooth overlapping curls
    d. prevent breaks or splits
    ____

16. Creating tension by forcing hair between the thumb and back of a comb when making pin curls is called:
    a. ribboning
    b. smoothing
    c. arcing
    d. placing
    ____

17. Pin curls sliced from a shaping and formed without lifting the hair from the head are:
    a. stem curls
    b. design curls
    c. carved curls
    d. ridge curls
    ____

18. Two rows of ridge curls placed on the side of a head are:
    a. ridge waves
    b. skip waves
    c. alternating waves
    d. clockwise waves
    ____

19. Pin curls that allow the hair to flow upward and downward are called stand-up curls or:
    a. cascade curls
    b. alternating curls
    c. C-shaped curls
    d. skip waves
    ____

20. Barrel curls are similar to a roller, but do not have the same:
    a. base
    b. tension
    c. volume
    d. angle ____

21. The panel of hair on which a roller is placed is the:
    a. stem
    b. section
    c. base
    d. subsection ____

22. Hair between the scalp and the first turn of a roller is the:
    a. curl
    b. base
    c. arc
    d. stem ____

23. For a roller set where little or no volume is required, the rollers should be placed:
    a. on-base
    b. off-base
    c. half-base
    d. down-base ____

24. The point where curls of opposite directions meet forming a recessed area is:
    a. indentation
    b. convex
    c. mobility
    d. directional ____

25. The metal edge of roller clips placed at an angle against the hair can cause:
    a. no tension
    b. long curls
    c. loose tension
    d. hair breakage ____

26. Combing small sections of hair from the ends toward the scalp creating a cushion or base is:
    a. back-combing
    b. combing sections
    c. comb-outs
    d. roller patterns ____

27. To smooth hair that is back-combed, the teeth of the comb or brush should be held at a:
    a. 15-degree angle
    b. 45-degree angle
    c. 90-degree angle
    d. 0-degree angle ____

28. When wrapping hair, very little volume will be attained provided the:
    a. style is correct
    b. hair at the scalp is not lifted
    c. hair is brushed smooth
    d. round brushes are used ____

29. The nozzle attachment used in blow-drying to create a steady stream of air is the:
    a. handle
    b. styling brush
    c. concentrator
    d. heating element ____

30. The tool attachment used to dry hair softly and accentuate the textural definition is a:
    a. diffuser
    b. nozzle
    c. concentrator
    d. texturizer
    ____

31. Teeth on a styling comb that are closely spaced remove curl definition and create a:
    a. textured surface
    b. shaped surface
    c. density surface
    d. smooth surface
    ____

32. Classic styling brushes having rows of round-tipped nylon bristles should be:
    a. heat sensitive and large
    b. heat resistant and antistatic
    c. heat resistant and narrow
    d. heat sensitive and heavy
    ____

33. An ideal brush for blow-drying fine hair quickly and adding lift to the scalp area is a:
    a. vent brush
    b. paddle brush
    c. grooming brush
    d. polish brush
    ____

34. A thickened liquid styling tool, spread with fingers, that creates the strongest control and distinct texture definition is:
    a. texturizer
    b. holding spray
    c. styling gel
    d. styling foam
    ____

35. A styling aid that holds fine hair with little or no heaviness is:
    a. heavy gel with weight
    b. holding spray
    c. texturizer
    d. pomade
    ____

36. A styling aid applied to damp wavy or curling hair to create a straight look when the hair is blow-dried is:
    a. styling foam
    b. straightening gel
    c. spray gel
    d. mousse
    ____

37. When blow-drying with a round brush, maximum lift is achieved by inserting the brush on base and directing the section up at a:
    a. slight angle
    b. back-and-forth motion
    c. 125-degree angle
    d. 45-degree angle
    ____

38. When using a concentrator to blow-dry straight or wavy hair, build the shape working from:
    a. left to right
    b. nape to crown
    c. top to bottom
    d. crown to sides
    ____

39. Waving and curling straight or pressed hair using special manipulative techniques on dry hair is:
    a. blow-drying
    b. thermal curling
    c. dry styling
    d. thermal rolling
    ____

40. The basic parts of a thermal iron are the rod handle, shell handle, and:
    a. barrel and shell
    b. heat regulator and stove
    c. bulb and barrel
    d. line handle and thermostat ____

41. The edge of a beveled flat iron that is nearest the stylist is the:
    a. inner edge
    b. control edge
    c. outer edge
    d. straight edge ____

42. To remove dirt, oils, and product residue from the barrel of a thermal iron, use a dampened towel with a soapy solution containing a few drops of:
    a. styling gel
    b. peroxide
    c. ammonia
    d. conditioner ____

43. Combs used with thermal irons should be about 7 inches long and made of:
    a. a flammable substance
    b. a plastic substance
    c. wide teeth
    d. a nonflammable substance ____

44. In thermal curling, hair is held at a 125-degree angle with medium tension and the curl is placed in the center if its base is a:
    a. full-base curl
    b. half-base curl
    c. thermal curl
    d. barrel curl ____

45. A type of thermal curl with only slight lift or volume can be achieved by using a 70-degree angle and:
    a. rolling hair completely off base
    b. rolling hair completely on base
    c. pushing the wave
    d. using liquid styling tools ____

46. A technique used to temporarily straighten extremely curly or unruly hair until the hair is shampooed is:
    a. hair pressing
    b. blow-drying
    c. thermal curling
    d. Velcro rollers ____

47. Applying a thermal pressing comb through the hair twice on each side to remove curl is a:
    a. hard press
    b. soft press
    c. thermal press
    d. medium press ____

48. Variations in hair texture are defined by the:
    a. length and style of the hair
    b. diameter and feel of the hair
    c. color and length of the hair
    d. color and style of the hair ____

49. Pressing wiry or curly hair requires more heat and pressure due to the:
    a. compact construction of the cuticle cells
    b. length and diameter of the cuticle cells
    c. diameter of the medulla cells
    d. texture and construction of the follicle cells ____

50. A tight scalp can be made more flexible with hair brushing and the systematic use of:
    a. conditioning masks
    b. scalp massage
    c. conditioning shampoos
    d. roller sets ____

51. The temperature of pressing combs should be tested:
    a. on a piece of light paper
    b. with running water
    c. on the client
    d. on a damp towel ____

52. To prevent the smoking or burning off of hair during the pressing treatment, avoid:
    a. excessive pressing oil
    b. excessive pressure
    c. excessive tension
    d. excessive pressing ____

53. When executing an updo, always inspect the shape you are building from every angle to determine:
    a. dimension and balance
    b. balance and proportion
    c. length and building
    d. texture and balance ____

54. A styling product available in a variety of strengths applied in the form of a mist to hold a style in position is:
    a. hair spray
    b. mousse
    c. foam
    d. liquid tools ____

55. A method of curling hair by winding a strand around a rod is a(n):
    a. pin curl
    b. on-base curl
    c. thermal curl
    d. spiral curl ____

CHAPTER 16—BRAIDING AND BRAID EXTENSIONS

1. In some African tribes, different styles of braiding signified a person's:
   a. personal bonds
   b. social status within the community
   c. fashion statement
   d. esthetic significance

   ____

2. Styling performed without chemicals or dyes and when the natural curl or coil pattern of hair is not altered is:
   a. traditional hairstyling
   b. natural hairstyling
   c. textured services
   d. unisex styling

   ____

3. To avoid misunderstandings in performing natural styling services, it is necessary to perform a(n):
   a. quality client consultation
   b. elaborate conditioning treatment
   c. excellent shampoo procedure
   d. preliminary scalp massage

   ____

4. When performing a consultation for natural hairstyling services, the focus should be on:
   a. service price
   b. time and effort
   c. hair length
   d. hair texture

   ____

5. In natural hairstyling services, texture refers to the diameter and feel of hair plus the:
   a. structure of hair
   b. condition of hair
   c. wave pattern
   d. length configuration

   ____

6. In textured hair, a coil configuration is defined as having a:
   a. square pattern
   b. tight curl pattern
   c. circular pattern
   d. loose curl pattern

   ____

7. To create length and soften facial lines with a square face, the hair should be styled with:
   a. waves and curls to create balance
   b. an updo style to create height
   c. a wave pattern to create depth
   d. a full style that frames the face

   ____

8. Styles with partial bangs or braids that frame the face and minimize a wide forehead should be used for facial shapes that are:
   a. round shaped
   b. an inverted triangle
   c. square shaped
   d. oval shaped

   ____

9. Hair with no previous coloring or lightening treatments, chemicals, or physical abuse is considered:
   a. chemical free hair
   b. textured hair
   c. structured hair
   d. natural or virgin

   ____

10. The brush recommended for scalp stimulation and removal of dirt and lint from locks is:
   a. vent brush
   b. boar-bristle brush
   c. nylon-bristle brush
   d. paddle brush

   ____

11. The bristles of a square paddle brush that are pneumatic will collapse when they encounter too much:
   a. resistance
   b. oil and dirt
   c. tension
   d. extension

   ____

12. The most important feature of a wide-toothed comb is the:
   a. distance between the teeth of the comb
   b. length of the comb handle
   c. colors available for the comb
   d. designs of the comb's teeth

   ____

13. A diffuser dries hair without disturbing the finished look or:
   a. dehydrating hair
   b. conditioning hair
   c. blending hair
   d. shortening hair

   ____

14. A manufactured synthetic fiber that does not reflect light and is similar in texture to extremely curly or coiled hair is:
   a. kanekalon
   b. yam
   c. nylon
   d. rayon

   ____

15. When curly hair is braided wet, it shrinks and recoils and may cause excess:
   a. matte finish
   b. slipping
   c. manufactured shine
   d. pulling and tension

   ____

16. To make straight or resistant hair more pliable when braiding, apply a:
   a. silicone shine spray
   b. light coat of wax or pomade
   c. heavy conditioner
   d. synthetic fiber

   ____

17. When blow-drying textured hair, the hair becomes soft and the wave pattern becomes:
   a. elongated
   b. sectioned
   c. combed
   d. tangled

   ____

18. The three-strand underhand braid technique where strands are woven under the center strand is a:
    a. twist braid
    b. visible braid
    c. inverted braid
    d. invisible braid ____

19. The three-strand braid produced by overlapping the strands on top of each other is the:
    a. inverted braid
    b. box braid
    c. micro-braid
    d. visible braid ____

20. The two-strand braid where the hair strands are twisted around each other is the:
    a. inverted braid
    b. fishtail braid
    c. rope braid
    d. visible braid ____

21. In the fishtail braid, hair is picked up from the sides and added to the strands:
    a. as often as necessary
    b. as they are crossed over each other
    c. to make a third strand
    d. as they are split over each other ____

22. Partings for braids can be square, triangular, or rectangular and determine:
    a. where the braid is placed and how it moves
    b. the length and direction of the finished braid
    c. the shape of the underhand or overhand technique
    d. the hair texture and where the braid is placed ____

23. Extensions for single braids are integrated into natural hair using the:
    a. two-strand overhand technique
    b. three-strand underhand technique
    c. individual braid technique
    d. medium to large techniques ____

24. Narrow, visible braids that lie close to the scalp created with a three-strand on-the-scalp braid technique are:
    a. french braids
    b. cornrows
    c. fishtail braids
    d. free-hanging braids ____

25. Extensions added to cornrows or individual braids with the feed-in method build the braid up:
    a. with excessive weight
    b. using tension
    c. three stands as once
    d. strand by strand ____

26. Natural textured hair intertwined and meshed together forming a single or separate network of hair is called:
    a. dreadlocks
    b. extensions
    c. cornrows
    d. braids ____

27. Three basic methods of hair locking are the comb technique, braids or extensions, and:
    a. networking
    b. meshing
    c. block rolling
    d. palm rolling ____

28. The gentle palm rolling method of locking hair takes advantage of the hair's natural:
    a. length and texture
    b. ability to grow
    c. texture and diameter
    d. ability to coil ____

29. The traditional cornrow is flat, natural, and:
    a. set in diagonal partings
    b. contoured to the scalp
    c. spiral in design
    d. overextended or misplaced ____

30. Synthetic hair fiber, human hair fiber, or yarn can be added to a single braid to form a:
    a. lock
    b. cornrow
    c. fishtail braid
    d. rope braid ____

CHAPTER 17—WIGS AND HAIR ENHANCEMENTS

1. The wig service costs and maintenance should be discussed during the:
   a. follow-up visit
   b. client consultation
   c. shampoo procedure
   d. fitting procedure ____

2. The artificial covering that covers 100 percent of the client's natural hair is a:
   a. toupee
   b. wig
   c. hairpiece
   d. braids ____

3. A small hair addition used to cover the top or crown of the head is a(n):
   a. braid
   b. extension
   c. hairpiece
   d. wig ____

4. The fastest way to determine whether a strand of hair is synthetic is to:
   a. burn it with a match
   b. ask the manufacturer
   c. shampoo the hair
   d. style the hair ____

5. With exposure, the color of human hair wigs may:
   a. last
   b. reset
   c. oxidize
   d. strengthen ____

6. Synthetic wigs that are particularly durable are made out of:
   a. silk
   b. polyester
   c. yak
   d. modacrylic ____

7. The most expensive wigs are constructed using:
   a. synthetic materials
   b. human hair
   c. monacrylic materials
   d. human hair mix ____

8. The root ends of hair with the cuticle placed in the same direction to prevent tangling is:
   a. human hair
   b. fallen hair
   c. tangle-free hair
   d. turned hair ____

9. A hand-knotted wig constructed for a secure fit with an elasticized mesh fiber base is a:
   a. connected weft
   b. cap wig
   c. capless wig
   d. synthetic wig ____

10. The hand-tied method of wig construction resembles actual hair growth with:
    a. flexibility at the root area
    b. availability in many colors
    c. ease of care
    d. special fitting requirements ____

11. A head-shaped form used for securing a wig is a:
    a. client
    b. form
    c. block
    d. canvas
    ____

12. When mounting a wig to a block, the wig should be pinned evenly using:
    a. bobby pins
    b. staples
    c. T-shaped pins
    d. H-shaped pins
    ____

13. When performing a haircutting procedure on a wig, the general goal is to make the wig:
    a. fit properly
    b. achieve weight
    c. shorter
    d. look realistic
    ____

14. When cutting a wig using a free-form method, move from longer to shorter lengths, working toward the:
    a. length
    b. weight
    c. sides
    d. form
    ____

15. Recommended styling products for wigs should be formulated for:
    a. color-treated hair
    b. natural hair
    c. textured hair
    d. synthetic hair
    ____

16. Before placing the wig on the head the hair should be:
    a. sectioned and secure
    b. flat and even
    c. wrapped and in rollers
    d. in pin curls and secure
    ____

17. When shampooing a wig, avoid shampoos that have a(n):
    a. oil base
    b. sulfur base
    c. conditioning base
    d. bolster base
    ____

18. Synthetic hair colors used on wigs and hairpieces are standardized using:
    a. natural color level ring
    b. black to red color ring
    c. 90 colors on the haircolor ring
    d. 70 colors on the haircolor ring
    ____

19. Prior to performing a color application on a wig or hairpiece, perform a:
    a. metallic test
    b. patch test
    c. strand test
    d. pulling test
    ____

20. Hairpieces with base openings that allow a client's hair to be pulled and blended are:
    a. full wig pieces
    b. weft base hairpieces
    c. interlocking hairpieces
    d. integration hairpieces
    ____

21. A small wig for men used to cover the top and crown of the head is a:
    a. toupee
    b. wraparound
    c. track
    d. weave
    ____

22. Hair additions secured to the base of natural hair that add length, volume, texture, or color are:
    a. manufactured wigs
    b. hair extensions
    c. hair wraps
    d. hair combs
    ____

23. Hair attached to an on-the-scalp braid that serves as the track is secured using a:
    a. track-and-sew method
    b. glue-and-blunt method
    c. track-and-angle method
    d. sew-and-diagonal method
    ____

24. When sewing an extension onto a track, the needle should be:
    a. dull and pointed
    b. straight and long
    c. sharp and dull
    d. straight or curved
    ____

25. The sewing stitch where the thread is wound around the needle twice is the:
    a. double-lock stitch
    b. secure lock stitch
    c. overcast stitch
    d. loop stitch
    ____

26. Attaching hair wefts or single strands with an adhesive or glue is a:
    a. track method
    b. lockstitch method
    c. sewing method
    d. bonding method
    ____

27. Hair that is bonded can be successfully shampooed provided it is done:
    a. gently
    b. often
    c. weekly
    d. monthly
    ____

28. The fusion method of extensions requires that the bonding material be activated with:
    a. bonding materials and no pressure
    b. wefts and pressure
    c. heat and finger pressure
    d. heat from a special tool
    ____

29. The fusion procedure involves wrapping both the client's hair and a:
    a. sectioned-based strip
    b. free-form strip
    c. keratin-based strip
    d. adhesive-based strip
    ____

30. A styling maintenance program educates clients in the use of:
    a. styling products
    b. client's budget
    c. health issues
    d. catalog prices
    ____

CHAPTER 18—CHEMICAL TEXTURE SERVICES

1. The chemical texture service that loosens overly curly hair into loose curls or waves is:
   a. curl softening
   b. curl re-formation
   c. alternate waving
   d. swelling compound ____

2. All chemical texture procedures involve changing the hair structure using:
   a. steady and constant changes
   b. chemical and layer changes
   c. physical and wave changes
   d. chemical and physical changes ____

3. The exterior hair structure layer that protects the hair from damage is the:
   a. cuticle
   b. medulla
   c. follicle
   d. shaft ____

4. The layer of the hair that provides strength and elasticity is the:
   a. medulla
   b. cortex
   c. regular
   d. arrector ____

5. Hair bonds that cannot be broken by heat or water are:
   a. disulfide bonds
   b. cuticle bonds
   c. sulfur bonds
   d. inner bonds ____

6. The natural pH of hair is between:
   a. 4.0 and 5.0
   b. 4.5 and 5.5
   c. 5.0 and 6.5
   d. 6.0 and 7.0 ____

7. One of the most important parts of a successful texture service is the:
   a. shampoo consultation
   b. client consultation
   c. draping procedure
   d. technical skill ____

8. Permanent waves cannot be performed if the hair is coated with:
   a. hydrogen shampoo
   b. metallic shine
   c. epsom salts
   d. metallic salts ____

9. Disulfide bonds are chemical-based side bonds that are formed when:
   a. three peptide bonds are broken apart
   b. sulfur atoms in two adjacent protein chains are joined together
   c. two salt-type chains are joined together
   d. three salt bonds are joined together ____

10. The measurement used to determine the hydrogen ions in a solution is:
    a. potential of hydrogen
    b. chemical composition
    c. potential negativity
    d. chemical solution ____

11. Chemical texturizers temporarily raise the pH of the hair by lifting the cuticle layer to:
    a. allow penetration to the medulla layer
    b. allow amino acids to swell
    c. allow penetration to the cortex layer
    d. allow keratin proteins to be removed ____

12. Long, coiled polypeptide chains that are part of the hairs structure are:
    a. salt bonds
    b. keratin proteins
    c. alkaline proteins
    d. peptide bonds ____

13. The client record card should include a complete evaluation of the length, texture, color, and:
    a. condition of the hair
    b. previous style of the hair
    c. client's favorite color
    d. the client's age ____

14. During the hair and scalp analysis procedure, the stylist should look for:
    a. cream conditioners
    b. abrasions or signs of scalp disease
    c. previous styling products used
    d. previous successful hair services ____

15. Hair texture that requires a longer processing or rewetting of solution to ensure complete saturation is:
    a. regular-textured hair
    b. fine-textured hair
    c. wavy-textured hair
    d. coarse-textured hair ____

16. The measurement of the number of hairs per square inch on the head is:
    a. density
    b. length
    c. porosity
    d. elasticity ____

17. An indication of the strength of the side bonds is:
    a. porosity
    b. elasticity
    c. flexibility
    d. absorption ____

18. The second process of a permanent wave is the:
    a. physical change process
    b. elasticity change process
    c. chemical change process
    d. influence change process ____

19. In permanent waving, the size of the curl is determined by the:
    a. position of the rod
    b. length of the hair
    c. wrapping of the rod
    d. size of the rod ____

20. The permanent wave rod that produces a uniform curl along the entire width of the strand is a:
    a. straight rod
    b. concave rod
    c. convex rod
    d. loop rod ____

21. A wrapping technique using two endpapers, one placed under the strand and one over is the:
    a. bookend wrap
    b. double-flat wrap
    c. single-flat wrap
    d. end wrap ____

22. Permanent wave rods are placed onto subsections of a panel called:
    a. base sections
    b. panel sections
    c. inverted sections
    d. center sections ____

23. The position of a permanent wave rod in relation to its base section is the:
    a. base direction
    b. rod angle
    c. wrapping angle
    d. base placement ____

24. The technique of wrapping at a 90-degree angle or straight out from the center is:
    a. half-off base placement
    b. base direction placement
    c. greater volume placement
    d. lesser volume placement ____

25. The two basic types of wrapping hair around a perm rod are the spiral method and:
    a. loop method
    b. croquignole method
    c. placement method
    d. horizontal method ____

26. A technique used to wrap extra-long hair using two rods in opposite directions is a(n):
    a. croquignole perm wrap
    b. ends perm wrap
    c. piggyback wrap
    d. spiral perm wrap ____

27. A reduction reaction involves either the addition of hydrogen or removal of:
    a. oxygen
    b. peroxide
    c. carbon
    d. nitrogen ____

28. A common, colorless reducing agent used in chemical texture services is:
    a. alkalizing agent
    b. thioglycolic acid
    c. reducing agent
    d. endothermic acid ____

29. The main reducing agent in alkaline permanents is:
    a. sodium hydroxide
    b. ammonium thioglycolate
    c. ammonium hydroxide
    d. ammonium bromide ____

30. Most alkaline permanent waves have a pH between:
    a. 9.0 and 9.6
    b. 9.0 and 10.1
    c. 8.0 and 10.0
    d. 9.5 and 10.1 ____

31. The primary low pH reducing agent in acid waves is:
    a. ammonium hydroxide
    b. glyceryl monothermic
    c. ammonium thioglycolate
    d. glyceryl monothioglycolate ____

32. An exothermic chemical reaction produces:
    a. thio
    b. heat
    c. hydrogen
    d. reactions ____

33. The basic components of acid waves are permanent wave solution and:
    a. conditioner and activator
    b. neutralizer and stabilizer
    c. activator and neutralizer
    d. shampoo and neutralizer ____

34. An endothermic wave must be activated using a(n):
    a. ammonia lotion
    b. outside heat source
    c. sulfite source
    d. reducing agent ____

35. In permanent waving, the processing should be determined by the:
    a. strength of the solution
    b. size of the rods
    c. processing time
    d. length of the hair ____

36. Hair that is too weak to hold a curl or may be completely straight after a perm is:
    a. overcurly
    b. over-processed
    c. oversaturated
    d. underprocessed ____

37. The process of stopping the action of a permanent wave is:
    a. rinsing
    b. rebuilding
    c. normalizing
    d. neutralization ____

38. Permanent wave solution should be rinsed from the hair for a minimum of:
    a. 2 minutes
    b. 10 minutes
    c. 5 minutes
    d. 15 minutes ____

39. A 90-degree perm wrap that minimizes stress and tension on the hair is:
    a. half off base
    b. on base
    c. overdirected
    d. curved base ____

40. The process of rearranging extremely curly hair into a straighter or smoother form is:
    a. chemical hair relaxing
    b. chemical smoothing
    c. continuation
    d. neutralizing ____

41. In extremely curly hair, the thinnest and weakest sections of the hair strand are located at the:
    a. twists
    b. roots
    c. diameter
    d. shaft ____

42. Thio chemical relaxers usually have a pH value above:
    a. 5
    b. 10
    c. 9
    d. 6 ____

43. The active ingredient in all hydroxide relaxers is the hydroxide:
    a. viscosity
    b. neutralization
    c. thio
    d. ion ____

44. All hydroxide relaxers can swell the hair up to:
    a. tenfold its normal diameter
    b. twice its normal diameter
    c. once its normal diameter
    d. three times its diameter ____

45. Hydroxide relaxers remove one atom of sulfur from a disulfide bond converting it into a:
    a. lanthionine bond
    b. hydrogen bond
    c. sulfur bond
    d. cross bond ____

46. Disulfide bonds broken by hydroxide relaxers can never be:
    a. restretched
    b. re-formed
    c. oxidized
    d. compatible ____

47. Hydroxide ions left in the hair after a relaxer can be neutralized using a(n):
    a. acid-balanced shampoo
    b. conditioning rinse
    c. thio neutralizer
    d. acid-free shampoo ____

48. Relaxers containing one component used without any additional mixing are:
    a. thio relaxers
    b. neutral relaxers
    c. metal hydroxide relaxers
    d. normalizing relaxers ____

49. Sodium hydroxide relaxers (NaOH) are commonly called:
    a. potassium relaxers
    b. lye relaxers
    c. thio relaxers
    d. guanidine relaxers ____

50. A relaxer with two components mixed immediately prior to use is:
    a. ammonium hydroxide relaxer
    b. guanidine hydroxide relaxer
    c. thioglycolate relaxer
    d. lithium hydroxide relaxer ____

51. Lithium hydroxide relaxers and potassium hydroxide relaxers are advertised and sold as:
    a. conditioner relaxers
    b. no-lye relaxers
    c. no chemical relaxers
    d. lye relaxers ____

52. Ammonium sulfite and ammonium bisulfite are marketed as:
    a. lanthionization relaxers
    b. mild alternative relaxers
    c. no-hydroxide relaxers
    d. lye relaxers ____

53. Cream used to protect the skin and scalp during a hair-relaxing process is:
    a. neutral cream
    b. scalp cream
    c. coating cream
    d. base cream ____

54. The strength of relaxers is determined by the concentration of:
    a. ammonia
    b. hydroxide
    c. salts
    d. atoms ____

55. To avoid overprocessing during a retouch relaxer application, wait until the last few minutes of processing to apply relaxer to the area:
    a. closest to the midshaft
    b. closest to the scalp
    c. closest to the sides
    d. closest to the front ____

56. Conditioners with an acidic pH that condition and normalize hair prior to shampooing are:
    a. conditioning rinses
    b. conditioning shampoos
    c. normalizing lotions
    d. acid-based relaxers ____

57. Curl re-formation does not straighten the hair, it simply makes the existing curl:
    a. larger and looser
    b. smaller and longer
    c. tighter and open
    d. open and soft ____

58. To avoid scalp irritation, prior to the application of a hydroxide relaxer never:
    a. shampoo the hair
    b. cut the hair
    c. condition the hair
    d. comb the hair ____

59. To avoid excessive stretching of the hair when combing out tangles, use a:
    a. tail comb
    b. plastic comb
    c. wide-toothed comb
    d. barber comb ____

60. Performing texture services involves powerful chemicals that must be handled with:
    a. ease
    b. caution
    c. gloves
    d. disregard
    ____

61. The term used to describe removing excess water before the application of a neutralizer is:
    a. processing
    b. conditioning
    c. blotting
    d. rinsing
    ____

62. When checking for test curl development, the test curl should reflect:
    a. loose S formation
    b. firm S formation
    c. small wave
    d. breakage
    ____

63. When performing test curls, the rod should be unwound approximately:
    a. ½ turn
    b. 1 turn
    c. 1½ turns
    d. 2 full turns
    ____

64. Incorrect placement of the rubber band of perm rods will cause band marks or:
    a. shrinkage
    b. protection
    c. tension
    d. breakage
    ____

65. When working with hair that has been chemically relaxed, you should avoid using:
    a. shampoo
    b. shears
    c. hot irons
    d. protective equipment
    ____

CHAPTER 19—HAIRCOLORING

1. A key factor in determining appropriate haircoloring services is understanding the client's:
   a. age
   b. motivation
   c. service
   d. style
   ____

2. Once a stylist demonstrates the ability to skillfully color a client's hair, the client will generally:
   a. remain loyal
   b. switch to a different stylist
   c. ask the stylist to remove the haircolor
   d. never return to the salon again
   ____

3. In choosing hair color for a client, a determining factor is the hair:
   a. natural style
   b. profession
   c. length
   d. structure
   ____

4. The layer of the hair that provides strength and elasticity is the:
   a. cortex layer
   b. cuticle layer
   c. follicle layer
   d. medulla layer
   ____

5. The outermost layer of the hair that protects and provides strength is the:
   a. cuticle layer
   b. medulla layer
   c. papilla layer
   d. structure layer
   ____

6. In individual hair strands, hair texture is determined by the:
   a. cuticle
   b. cortex
   c. diameter
   d. length
   ____

7. Hair color applied to fine hair may look:
   a. darker
   b. lighter
   c. shorter
   d. dull
   ____

8. Haircoloring services on coarse-textured hair may take:
   a. faster to process
   b. longer to process
   c. porosity to process
   d. liquids to process
   ____

9. Hair with a tight cuticle resistant to moisture or chemicals is defined as having:
   a. average porosity
   b. poor porosity
   c. low porosity
   d. porous porosity
   ____

10. The predominant melanin that gives black or brown color to hair is:
    a. pheomelanin
    b. natural melanin
    c. individual melanin
    d. eumelanin
    ____

11. Pigment that lies under the natural hair color is the:
    a. contributing pigment
    b. combination pigment
    c. predominant pigment
    d. exposed pigment ____

12. The lightness or darkness of a color is called the:
    a. range
    b. level
    c. pigment
    d. degree ____

13. The system used by colorists to analyze the lightness or darkness of a hair color is the:
    a. measurement system
    b. natural system
    c. color system
    d. level system ____

14. Hair color levels are arranged on a scale from:
    a. 1 to 12
    b. 1 to 10
    c. 1 to 5
    d. 0 to 10 ____

15. Hair color tones can be described as:
    a. warm, neutral, and hot
    b. warm, neutral, and cool
    c. cool, neutral, and even
    d. cool, warm, and primary ____

16. Colors that absorb light and appear darker than their actual level are:
    a. primary colors
    b. cool colors
    c. warm colors
    d. neutral colors ____

17. Warm tones reflect light and may appear:
    a. ash
    b. smokey
    c. cool
    d. lighter ____

18. Colors that are described as sandy or tan are considered:
    a. primary tones
    b. natural tones
    c. intensity tones
    d. formulation tones ____

19. The first step in performing a haircolor service is to identify:
    a. the natural growth pattern
    b. natural levels
    c. neutral tones
    d. intensity tones ____

20. Colors that we see are contained in the:
    a. invisible light spectrum
    b. color wheel
    c. color formulation
    d. visible light spectrum ____

21. Artificial hair colors are developed from the primary and secondary colors that form:
    a. base colors
    b. tonality colors
    c. permanent tones
    d. drastic colors ____

22. A color that will help minimize orange tones in the hair is a:
    a. violet base color
    b. blue base color
    c. secondary color
    d. gold base color
    ____

23. A system that is used to understand color relationships is the:
    a. color wheel
    b. level system
    c. law of color
    d. primary color system
    ____

24. Colors that are pure or fundamental and cannot be achieved from a mixture are:
    a. level colors
    b. secondary colors
    c. cool colors
    d. primary colors
    ____

25. The primary colors are:
    a. red, blue, and orange
    b. blue, red, and violet
    c. yellow, blue, and red
    d. red, yellow, and green
    ____

26. The darkest and only cool primary color is:
    a. green
    b. ash
    c. red
    d. blue
    ____

27. Red added to blue-based colors will cause them to appear:
    a. lighter
    b. darker
    c. golden
    d. yellow
    ____

28. A color achieved by mixing a secondary color and its neighboring primary color is a:
    a. primary color
    b. tertiary color
    c. secondary color
    d. base color
    ____

29. Equal proportions of primary colors will produce:
    a. neutral
    b. secondary
    c. black
    d. brighter
    ____

30. A secondary color is obtained by mixing equal parts of two:
    a. base colors
    b. primary colors
    c. neutral colors
    d. cool colors
    ____

31. A primary and secondary color positioned opposite each other on the color wheel are:
    a. neutralizing colors
    b. combination colors
    c. opposing colors
    d. complementary colors
    ____

32. Complementary colors are used in color formulation to:
    a. oppose together
    b. attract each other
    c. neutralize each other
    d. highlight each other
    ____

33. The process of diffusing natural color pigment or artificial color from the hair is:
    a. hair lightening
    b. hair lifting
    c. hair tinting
    d. hair colorization ____

34. All permanent hair color products and lighteners contain an oxidizing agent and a(n):
    a. neutralizing agent
    b. developer ingredient
    c. alkalizing ingredient
    d. booster agent ____

35. A hair-lightening process occurs when the alkaline peroxide:
    a. breaks up the primary color
    b. breaks up the melanin
    c. dissolves the oxidizing agent
    d. breaks up the neutral color ____

36. Temporary color pigment molecules do not penetrate because they are:
    a. weak
    b. soft
    c. neutral
    d. large ____

37. Semipermanent hair color on average should last:
    a. 4 to 6 days
    b. 4 to 6 weeks
    c. 8 to 10 weeks
    d. 5 to 10 weeks ____

38. Haircoloring that penetrates the hair shaft and is formulated to deposit but not lift color is:
    a. demipermanent hair color
    b. permanent hair color
    c. semipermanent color
    d. semitemporary color ____

39. Demipermanent hair color is available in a variety of formulas including:
    a. creams, liquid, and sprays
    b. gels, creams, and lotions
    c. creams. gels, and liquid
    d. gels, powders, and sprays ____

40. Uncolored dye precursors that can be diffused into the hair shaft are used in ;
    a. gel hair color formulas
    b. permanent hair color formulas
    c. semipermanent hair color formulas
    d. temporary hair color formulas ____

41. Dye precursors that combine with hydrogen peroxide to form larger tint molecules are:
    a. aniline peroxide
    b. aniline derivatives
    c. base derivatives
    d. no-ammonia formulas ____

42. Although many semipermanent and demipermanent colors use alkalizing agents other than ammonia, they are not necessarily any less:
    a. damaging
    b. effective
    c. colorful
    d. durable ____

43. Permanent haircoloring products are mixed with:
    a. no-ammonia
    b. aniline derivates
    c. hydrogen peroxide
    d. dye precursors ____

44. Permanent hair color products used for gray hair remove natural pigment and:
    a. add natural pigment
    b. add artificial color
    c. remove gray hair
    d. add ammonia tint ____

45. To provide maximum lift in a one-process color service, most high-lift colors require:
    a. 20 volume peroxide
    b. 15 volume peroxide
    c. 30 volume peroxide
    d. 40 volume peroxide ____

46. Haircoloring products that change hair color by creating a progressive buildup contain:
    a. henna colors
    b. chemical colors
    c. metallic colors
    d. vegetable colors ____

47. The most common developer used in haircoloring is:
    a. chemical agent
    b. developer strength
    c. hydrogen peroxide
    d. compound agents ____

48. Lighteners are chemical compounds that lighten natural hair pigment by dispersing, dissolving, and:
    a. decreasing
    b. developer
    c. decolorizing
    d. achieving ____

49. When hydrogen peroxide is mixed with a lightener formula, it releases:
    a. volume
    b. oxygen
    c. color
    d. hydrogen ____

50. During the decolorization process, natural hair can go through as many as:
    a. 2 stages
    b. 1 stage
    c. 5 stages
    d. 10 stages ____

51. Toners are used to achieve pale, delicate colors and are applied to create the correct degree of:
    a. unwanted pigment
    b. contributing pigment
    c. gold pigment
    d. desired shade ____

52. The test required by the U.S. Federal Food, Drug and Cosmetic Act to determine client allergies or sensitivities is the:
    a. swab test
    b. process test
    c. strand test
    d. predisposition test ____

53. To determine how hair will react to a selected color formula, perform a(n):
    a. preliminary strand test
    b. predisposition test
    c. allergy test
    d. patch test ____

54. When selecting a semipermanent color, remember that color applied on top of color creates:
    a. a lighter color
    b. a natural color
    c. a darker color
    d. a brighter color ____

55. Permanent hair color applications are classified as double-process or:
    a. lifting processes
    b. single-process
    c. deposit colors
    d. strand processes ____

56. The application process that is used for first-time color applications is:
    a. retouch process
    b. double-process
    c. virgin application
    d. new application ____

57. Overlapping color can cause breakage and create a sign of roots or:
    a. lightening agent
    b. line of demarcation
    c. barrier line
    d. streaking ____

58. Double-process lightening is prelightening hair to a very blonde stage and applying a:
    a. toner
    b. foundation
    c. rinse
    d. bleach ____

59. For a single-process color for virgin hair, the color processes fastest at:
    a. the shaft
    b. the scalp
    c. the ends
    d. the middle ____

60. Cream lighteners are formulated to be used:
    a. with glaze
    b. on the scalp
    c. on the ends
    d. off the scalp ____

61. The three forms of hair lighteners are:
    a. cream, powder, and scalp
    b. oil, cream, and clear
    c. powder, conditioning, and oil
    d. oil, powder, and cream ____

62. An oxidizer added to hydrogen peroxide to increase its lifting power action is a(n):
    a. powder
    b. activator
    c. ion
    d. crystal
    ____

63. A technique of coloring strands of hair darker than the natural color is:
    a. highlighting
    b. double-process
    c. tinting
    d. lowlighting
    ____

64. A foil technique where a straight and narrow section of hair at the scalp is positioned for color or lightener application is:
    a. the cap technique
    b. slicing
    c. weaving
    d. lowlights
    ____

65. In the foil technique when selected strands are picked up from a narrow section of hair with a zigzag motion of the comb, and lightener is applied in:
    a. slicing
    b. baliage
    c. free-form technique
    d. weaving
    ____

66. When coloring for a client with 80 to 100 percent gray, the color levels that provide the best coverage are:
    a. level 8 or lighter
    b. level 9 or lighter
    c. level 4 and darker
    d. level 7 and darker
    ____

67. To cover unpigmented hair in a salt-and-pepper client, the color formulation should be:
    a. one level darker than the natural level
    b. two levels lighter than the natural level
    c. one level lighter than the natural level
    d. one shade darker than the desired level
    ____

68. Pretreating gray or very resistant hair to allow for better penetration is:
    a. formulating
    b. unpigmenting
    c. predisposition
    d. presoftening
    ____

69. Preparations designed to equal porosity and deposit a base color in one application are:
    a. neutralizers
    b. fillers
    c. stabilizers
    d. conditioners
    ____

70. To increase the longevity of a professional color service and preserve the health of clients' hair, the stylist should encourage them to use only:
    a. inexpensive products
    b. imported products
    c. professional products
    d. consumer products
    ____

CHAPTER 20—SKIN DISEASES AND DISORDERS

1. The signs of aging are influenced by factors such as the sun, health habits, lifestyle, and:
   a. water
   b. heredity
   c. vitamins
   d. oxygen ____

2. The percentage of skin aging that is caused by the rays of the sun is approximately:
   a. 50 to 55 percent
   b. 60 to 65 percent
   c. 70 to 75 percent
   d. 80 to 85 percent ____

3. The UV rays of the sun reach the skin in two different forms, which are:
   a. UVA and UVB rays
   b. VBC and ABA rays
   c. UVA and ULB rays
   d. UVB and ABB rays ____

4. The UVA rays that are deep-penetrating and can go through a glass window are:
   a. sun rays
   b. aging rays
   c. light rays
   d. ultra rays ____

5. Wrinkling and sagging of the skin are caused by weakening collagen fibers and:
   a. protein fibers
   b. tissue fibers
   c. elastin fibers
   d. dermis fibers ____

6. UVB rays contribute to the body's synthesis of vitamin D and other important:
   a. absorption
   b. minerals
   c. elements
   d. rejuvenation ____

7. Daily moisturizers or protective lotions should have a sunscreen with an SPF of at least:
   a. 5
   b. 8
   c. 10
   d. 15 ____

8. The American Cancer Society checklist used to recognize skin cancer is:
   a. asymmetry, big, colored, diameter
   b. border, color, diameter, evolving
   c. angle, border, continued, diameter
   d. asymmetry, border, color, diameter ____

9. A salon should not service a client who is suffering from a(n):
   a. skin condition
   b. inflamed skin disorder
   c. skin discoloration
   d. pustule ____

10. A small circumscribed elevation of the skin that contains no fluid but may develop pus is a:
    a. macula
    b. scar
    c. mole
    d. papule ____

11. An abnormal cell mass resulting from excessive multiplication of cells and varying in size, shape, and color is a:
    a. tumor
    b. mole
    c. macula
    d. bulla ____

12. A crack in the skin that penetrates the dermis is a:
    a. split
    b. crust
    c. pustule
    d. fissure ____

13. Keratin-filled cysts that appear just under the epidermis and have no visible openings are:
    a. milia
    b. ulcers
    c. crust
    d. pustules ____

14. Any thin plate of dry or oily epidermal flakes in the scalp area is referred to as:
    a. scales
    b. dandruff
    c. flakes
    d. comedo ____

15. Sebum from a comedo exposed to the environment turns black and:
    a. closes
    b. opens
    c. oxidizes
    d. removes ____

16. Comedones should be removed under aseptic conditions using proper:
    a. skin lotions
    b. extraction procedures
    c. electric tools
    d. skin conditioners ____

17. A chronic skin condition characterized by inflammation of the sebaceous glands is:
    a. freckles
    b. acne
    c. tumors
    d. milia ____

18. An inflammation of the sebaceous glands characterized by dry or oily crusting or itchiness is:
    a. seborrheic dermatitis
    b. seborrheic acne
    c. sebaceous masses
    d. bacterium acne ____

19. A dry, scaly skin condition due to a deficiency or absence of sebum caused by old age or exposure to the cold is:
    a. cystic
    b. cortisone
    c. rosacea
    d. asteatosis ____

20. A disorder of the sweat gland caused by excessive exposure to the heat is:
    a. steatoma
    b. miliaria rubra
    c. anhidrosis
    d. dermatitis ____

21. A painful itching skin disease with dry or moist lesions that a physician needs to treat is:
    a. eczema
    b. acne
    c. psoriasis
    d. cyst ____

22. A contagious recurring viral infection characterized by blisters on the lips or nostrils is:
    a. eczema simplex
    b. macula simplex
    c. herpes simplex
    d. contact dermatitis ____

23. The medical term for abnormal skin inflammation is:
    a. abrasion
    b. dermatitis
    c. psoriasis
    d. bulla ____

24. Prolonged or repeated direct skin contact with chemicals has the potential to cause:
    a. allergic reactions
    b. histamine reactions
    c. keloids
    d. absorption ____

25. The chemicals released by the immune system to enlarge the vessels around an injury are:
    a. correctors
    b. irritants
    c. allergens
    d. histamines ____

26. Surprisingly, a very common salon irritant is:
    a. soap
    b. air
    c. tap water
    d. shampoo ____

27. Abnormal brown or wine-colored skin discoloration with a circular and irregular shape is a:
    a. mole
    b. stain
    c. chloasma
    d. lentigo ____

28. The absence of melanin pigment from the body and skin sensitivity to light are signs of:
    a. nevus
    b. lentignes
    c. asteatosis
    d. albinism ____

29. A spot or blemish spot on the skin that requires medical attention if there is a change is a:
    a. blemish
    b. mole
    c. freckle
    d. keratoma ____

30. The most common type of skin cancer characterized by light or pearly nodules is:
    a. basal cell carcinoma
    b. malignant melanoma
    c. squamous cell melanoma
    d. verruca cell

____

CHAPTER 21—HAIR REMOVAL

1. Hair removal approaches fall into two major categories, which are:
   a. laser and waxing
   b. temporary and permanent
   c. waxing and tweezing
   d. permanent and semipermanent ____

2. Terms that refer to the overgrowth of hair on the body are hypertrichosis and:
   a. excessive
   b. hypersensitive
   c. hirsuties
   d. downy ____

3. During the client consultation, all clients should complete a questionnaire that discloses skin disorders, allergies, and:
   a. medications
   b. topicals
   c. diet
   d. assessments ____

4. One of the main purposes of a client consultation is to determine the presence of any:
   a. density
   b. follicles
   c. electrolysis
   d. contraindications ____

5. The removal of hair with electrical current that destroys the growth cells of the hair is:
   a. photoepilation
   b. electrolysis
   c. electromagnetic
   d. laser ____

6. Intense light therapy used to destroy the growth cells of the hair follicles is:
   a. photoepilation
   b. epilation
   c. electrolysis
   d. depilation ____

7. A rapid method of removing hair with the use of beams pulsed on the skin is:
   a. laser hair removal
   b. electromagnetic
   c. electrolysis
   d. photobeams ____

8. An absolute requirement for laser hair removal is that the hair being removed must be:
   a. lighter than the surrounding skin
   b. darker than the surrounding skin
   c. administered to the surrounding skin
   d. removed slowly ____

9. In the nape area, the most common form of hair removal is usually performed using electric:
   a. tweezers
   b. clippers
   c. shears
   d. lasers ____

10. A positive impact on the overall attractiveness of the face can be achieved with:
    a. evenly spaced eyes
    b. client consultation
    c. client's wishes
    d. correctly shaped eyebrows ____

11. The natural arch of the eyebrow follows the:
    a. orbital bone
    b. frontal bone
    c. mandible bone
    d. frontal muscle ____

12. A term used to describe unwanted hair is:
    a. downy hair
    b. lanugo hair
    c. papilla
    d. superfluous hair ____

13. Electronic tweezers transmit radio frequency energy into the follicle area, dehydrating and eventually destroying the:
    a. cuticle
    b. cortex
    c. lanugo
    d. papilla ____

14. A caustic substance used for the temporary removal of superfluous hair at the skin level is:
    a. a cold wax
    b. a photoepilation
    c. a depilatory
    d. electric tweezers ____

15. The product composition of cold and hot wax is primarily beeswax and:
    a. aloe gel
    b. resins
    c. sugar
    d. caustic ____

16. Disposable gloves should be worn during a waxing service to prevent contact with possible:
    a. inflamed skin
    b. sensitive skin
    c. previously treated skin
    d. bloodborne pathogens ____

17. Wax should never be applied over warts, moles, abrasions, or:
    a. irritated or inflamed skin
    b. dark or red areas
    c. freckles
    d. scaly skin ____

18. To prevent wax contamination, an applicator should be placed in the wax:
    a. twice
    b. once
    c. when needed
    d. often ____

19. In a waxing treatment, the wax should be applied:
    a. against the hair growth
    b. in the excessive amounts required
    c. in the direction of the hair growth
    d. in the treated areas ____

20. An epilator treatment that involves using a thick-based product appropriate for sensitive skin is:
    a. beeswax
    b. sugaring
    c. cold wax
    d. depilatory
    ____

21. Apply pressure to remove a fabric waxing strip and pull:
    a. straight up
    b. in the direction of hair growth
    c. downward
    d. in the opposite direction of hair growth
    ____

22. To prevent skin irritation or burns, the temperature of wax should be tested:
    a. on the client's skin
    b. prior to application
    c. after the application
    d. during the application
    ____

23. A temporary hair removal method practiced in many Eastern cultures is the process of:
    a. threading
    b. tattooing
    c. removal
    d. laser
    ____

24. If redness or swelling occurs after a waxing treatment, soothe the skin with the application of:
    a. aloe gel
    b. lotion
    c. disinfectant
    d. astringent
    ____

25. A wax that is thick and does not require fabric strips for removal is:
    a. aloe wax
    b. cold wax
    c. honey wax
    d. chemical wax
    ____

CHAPTER 22—FACIALS

1. The preliminary parts of a facial treatment that determine the treatments to be performed are:
   a. skin consultation and payment
   b. skin analysis and consultation
   c. client consultation and draping
   d. skin analysis and product choice ____

2. The health screening performed prior to a facial treatment is used by the technician to determine any:
   a. product preference
   b. client lifestyle
   c. financial background
   d. contraindications ____

3. Clients with obvious skin abnormalities such as open sores, fever blisters, or abnormal-looking signs should be:
   a. advised of services
   b. provided treatments
   c. referred to a physician
   d. provided free services ____

4. When removing a cleanser from the eye area, it should be removed with damp facial sponges or cotton pads:
   a. in an upward and outward movement
   b. in down and across movements
   c. with friction movements
   d. in upward and across movements ____

5. When performing a skin analysis with a magnifying lamp, the first thing the technician should look for is the presence or absence of:
   a. skin types
   b. visible pores
   c. evaporated cells
   d. oily skin areas ____

6. If the client is not producing enough sebum, the skin type is characterized as:
   a. clean
   b. oily
   c. alipidic
   d. normal ____

7. Skin that has small pores and may be flaky or dry with fine lines and wrinkles is characterized as:
   a. dehydrated
   b. oily
   c. normal
   d. sensitive ____

8. Oily skin or skin that produces too much sebum may appear shiny or greasy and have:
   a. dead cells
   b. small pores
   c. flakes
   d. large pores ____

9. Pores that are clogged from dead cells building up in the follicle may have the appearance of open:
   a. creams
   b. comedones
   c. milia
   d. sebum ____

10. The difference between closed and open comedones is the size of the follicle opening or the:
   a. gland
   b. sebum
   c. ostium
   d. skin ____

11. When the follicle becomes clogged, resulting in an infection of the follicle, it is caused by a type of acne bacteria called:
   a. hydrators
   b. anaerobic
   c. sebum imbalance
   d. hyperpigmentation ____

12. Red pimples that do not have a pus head are referred to as:
   a. elastin pimples
   b. acne papules
   c. acne pigmentation
   d. acne oxygen ____

13. A skin condition caused by sun exposure or hormone imbalances resulting in dark blotches of color in areas of the skin is:
   a. hypertrichosis
   b. hydrators
   c. dehydration
   d. hyperpigmentation ____

14. A chronic hereditary disorder indicated by constant or frequent facial blushing is:
   a. rosacea
   b. tinea
   c. pustules
   d. comedones ____

15. A nonfoaming cleansing product that is designed to cleanse dry and sensitive skin is:
   a. astringent lotion
   b. cleansing powder
   c. foaming cleanser
   d. cleansing milk ____

16. Cleansing products that foam and rinse off easily generally contain surfactants also known as:
   a. astringents
   b. skin toners
   c. detergents
   d. exfoliants ____

17. Skin products designed to lower the pH of skin after cleansing and remove excess cleansing product are fresheners, astringents, or:
   a. detergents
   b. surfactants
   c. toners
   d. emollients ____

18. Exfoliant products are used on skin surfaces to make the skin look smoother by:
    a. removing excess moisture
    b. removing excess dead cells
    c. removing makeup
    d. adding moisture to skin

    ____

19. Cosmetology professionals are only allowed to use products that remove surface dead cells from the:
    a. internal dermis
    b. stratum corneum
    c. stratum dermis
    d. dermal layer

    ____

20. A gentle chemical exfoliation acid that helps dissolve the bonds and intercellular cement between cells is:
    a. alpha hydroxy acid
    b. emulsion acid
    c. astringent acid
    d. steaming acid

    ____

21. A salon-type of alpha hydroxy acid exfoliant that contains a concentration of 20 to 30 percent acid is referred to as a:
    a. skin brushing
    b. peel
    c. beta hydroxy acid
    d. removal

    ____

22. A chemical exfoliant that works by dissolving keratin protein in the surface skin cells is known as an enzyme peel or:
    a. keratolytic
    b. salt peel
    c. cream treatment
    d. tonic peel

    ____

23. An enzyme cream-type skin peel that forms a crust and is rolled off the skin is a:
    a. papain
    b. scrubbing
    c. emulsion
    d. gommage

    ____

24. Moisturizers that increase the water content of the skin's surface with a product that is water-binding are known as:
    a. toners
    b. astringents
    c. hydrators
    d. emollients

    ____

25. A fatty or oily ingredient used to block moisture from leaving the skin is a(n):
    a. emollient
    b. exfoliant
    c. toner
    d. sunscreen

    ____

26. Clients should be advised to use sunscreens that protect against both UVA and:
    a. VBB sun rays
    b. UVB sun rays
    c. UTB sun rays
    d. ATB sun rays

    ____

27. Highly concentrated skin products applied under a moisturizer or sunscreen are:
    a. serums
    b. tonics
    c. masks
    d. shielding ____

28. Lubricants applied to the face to make the skin slippery during a treatment are:
    a. exfoliant creams
    b. massage creams
    c. AHA
    d. clay masks ____

29. Soothing masks that have antibacterial ingredients and are helpful for acne-prone skin are:
    a. water based
    b. medicated based
    c. moisture based
    d. clay based ____

30. Masks that do not dry the skin and often contain oils and emollients as well as humectants are:
    a. oil masks
    b. gel masks
    c. cream masks
    d. serums ____

31. Paraffin used as a mask has no skin benefit unless mixed with a(n):
    a. exfoliating cream
    b. treatment cream
    c. oxygen cream
    d. massage treatment ____

32. A plaster-like mask that, when mixed with water, causes a chemical reaction is known as a(n):
    a. clay mask
    b. alginate mask
    c. quick mask
    d. modelage mask ____

33. The thin, open-meshed, woven cotton fabric used in the penetration of the mask application is:
    a. plastic
    b. silk
    c. gauze
    d. satin ____

34. The term used to describe the manual or mechanical manipulation of the body is:
    a. friction
    b. massage
    c. movements
    d. circulation ____

35. To master massage techniques, the cosmetologist should have a basic working knowledge of:
    a. anatomy and physiology
    b. costs of products
    c. skin toners
    d. gommage ____

36. The direction of movement in massage techniques should always be from the insertion of the muscle:
    a. toward the end
    b. behind the muscle
    c. toward its origin
    d. at the motor point ____

37. The massage movement that is a light continuous stroking movement with the fingers in a slow rhythmic manner is:
    a. tapotement
    b. petrissage
    c. kneading
    d. effleurage ____

38. The kneading massage movement performed by lifting, squeezing, and pressing the tissue with light, firm pressure is:
    a. petrissage
    b. rolling
    c. effleurage
    d. stroking ____

39. The deep rubbing of friction massage movements on the skin has been known to have a significant effect on the:
    a. texture and appearance of dry skin
    c. activity and texture of the skin
    b. circulation and glandular activity of the skin
    d. underlying structure activity of the skin ____

40. The most stimulating type of massage that should be performed using extreme care and discretion is:
    a. fulling
    b. stroking
    c. tapotement
    d. chucking ____

41. The point on the skin over the muscle where pressure and stimulation will cause contraction of the muscle is referred to as the:
    a. insertion point
    b. motor point
    c. origin point
    d. connection point ____

42. A significant benefit of a facial steamer that heats and produces steam is that the steam produced will soften and relax:
    a. dry skin conditions
    b. oily skin conditions
    c. follicle accumulations
    d. the client ____

43. When using the brushing machine to perform an exfoliation, the skin should be treated with a(n):
    a. thin layer of cleanser or moisturizer
    b. fairly thick layer of cleanser or moisturizer
    c. face freshener
    d. astringent lotion ____

44. The skin suction and cold spray machine is used to increase circulation and should be used only on nonsensitive or:
    a. oily skin
    b. hydrated skin
    c. mature skin
    d. noninflamed skin ____

45. The use of electric currents to treat the skin is a form of:
    a. electrotherapy
    b. magnetic therapy
    c. cold spray therapy
    d. microfarad therapy ____

46. The process of softening and emulsifying hardened sebum stuck in the follicles is called:
    a. massage therapy
    b. passive therapy
    c. desincrustation
    d. shock treatments ____

47. Water-soluble products are penetrated into the skin using galvanic current and a process called:
    a. penetration
    b. iontophoresis
    c. active anode
    d. extraction ____

48. A galvanic treatment using a computerized device to tone skin and produce a lifting effect on aging skin is:
    a. microcurrent
    b. microwaves
    c. galvanic imaging
    d. Tesla currents ____

49. The therapeutic use of essential oils to enhance a person's physical and emotional well-being is:
    a. retailing
    b. consultations
    c. antidepressants
    d. aromatherapy ____

50. After the first treatment, every new client should be provided with a thorough consultation that consists of salon treatment programs, education, and:
    a. positive effects
    b. verbal instructions
    c. proper home care
    d. prescription medication ____

CHAPTER 23—FACIAL MAKEUP

1. A base makeup that is used to cover or even out the coloring of skin is:
   a. blush
   b. roll-on
   c. foundation
   d. cream ____

2. Foundation bases are available in stick, cream, mineral powder, and:
   a. foam
   b. roll-on
   c. tint
   d. liquid ____

3. Natural derived pigments or color agents added to foundations to provide color are:
   a. lakes
   b. minerals
   c. emollients
   d. liquids ____

4. The recommended foundation for light coverage on oily to combination skin is:
   a. water based
   b. oil free
   c. cream foundations
   d. natural foundations ____

5. Foundations that provide a heavier base coverage for dry skin are:
   a. water-based foundations
   b. cream foundations
   c. powder-type foundations
   d. tinted base foundations ____

6. Foundation should be blended using:
   a. lint-free tissues
   b. disposable makeup sponge
   c. cotton cloths
   d. professional brush ____

7. Concealers that are used to hide dark circles and imperfections contain talc or:
   a. tint
   b. oil
   c. pigment
   d. silicone ____

8. To keep pressed powder in a cake form, it is usually blended with:
   a. mineral oil
   b. binding agents
   c. scented particles
   d. cornstarch agents ____

9. A makeup product primarily used to add a natural glow to the cheek or face area is a:
   a. blush
   b. foundation
   c. concealer
   d. highlight ____

10. Generally, a darker shade of eye color makes the natural color of the iris appear:
    a. darker
    b. closer
    c. lighter
    d. neutral
    ____

11. Color applied over the eye area to even out skin tones and provide a smooth surface for the blending of other colors is a:
    a. neutral color
    b. contour color
    c. medium color
    d. base color
    ____

12. A color in any finish that deepens and darkens the skin tone and minimizes a specific area is a:
    a. desired color
    b. contour color
    c. highlight color
    d. neutral color
    ____

13. To avoid infection in the tear duct or permanent pigmentation of the mucous membrane lining, eye pencils should never be used:
    a. on the outer rim of eyes
    b. near the lash area
    c. on the inner rim of eyes
    d. on the upper lids
    ____

14. A cosmetic preparation used to darken, define, and thicken eyelashes is:
    a. blush
    b. mascara
    c. foundation
    d. eye shadow
    ____

15. To clean professional makeup brushes, a gentle shampoo or brush solvent is used, and the brush is placed into running water with the:
    a. bristles being flat
    b. ferrule pointing upward
    c. ferrule pointing downward
    d. bristles being covered
    ____

16. Colors obtained by mixing equal parts of two primary colors are:
    a. tertiary colors
    b. complementary colors
    c. mixing colors
    d. secondary colors
    ____

17. A primary and secondary color directly opposite each other on the color wheel are:
    a. secondary colors
    b. conflicting colors
    c. complementary colors
    d. primary colors
    ____

18. Three main factors to consider when choosing color for a client are the client's hair color,
    a. eye color, and skin color
    b. eye placement, and skin texture
    c. skin color, and texture
    d. eye color, and results
    ____

19. Colors that are dominated by blues, greens, violets, and blue-reds are classified as:
    a. cool colors
    b. magenta colors
    c. complementary colors
    d. pigment colors ____

20. Skin tones that contain equal amounts of warm and cool colors are considered:
    a. basic skin tones
    b. neutral skin tones
    c. cool skin tones
    d. warm skin tones ____

21. Complementary colors for green eyes are brown-based reds, which include:
    a. green, blue, and silver
    b. copper, plum, and mauve
    c. taupe, caramel, and peach
    d. yellow, reds, and neutrals ____

22. The best type of lighting for color selection in the salon consultation area is:
    a. bright light
    b. natural light
    c. fluorescent light
    d. cool light ____

23. Foundation application should start at the center of the face and blend with:
    a. upward and outside motions
    b. outward and fast motions
    c. downward and slow motions
    d. outward and downward motions ____

24. A basic rule of makeup application is that highlighting emphasizes a feature and shadowing:
    a. minimizes a feature
    b. shades a feature
    c. maximizes a feature
    d. outlines a feature ____

25. The second portion of an oval-shaped type face is measured from the:
    a. hairline to the top of the eyebrows
    b. end of the nose to the bottom of the chin
    c. top of eyebrows to end of nose
    d. side of ears to end of nose ____

26. The facial shape composed of comparatively straight lines, a wide forehead, and square jaw is the:
    a. square-shaped face
    b. round-shaped face
    c. oval-shaped face
    d. diamond-shaped face ____

27. The long, narrow facial shape with greater length in proportion to its width is the:
    a. triangle-shaped face
    b. diamond-shaped face
    c. oblong-shaped face
    d. square-shaped face ____

28. To minimize a short, flat nose, a lighter foundation is applied:
    a. on the cheeks and sides of the nose, ending at the tip
    b. down the center of the nose, ending at the tip
    c. on the sides of the nose and nostrils
    d. onto the sides of the nose and into the laugh lines of the face

    ____

29. To set foundation and prevent the transfer to clothing, use:
    a. darker foundation
    b. translucent powder
    c. natural skin tones
    d. pressed powder

    ____

30. In eyebrow arching, the highest part of an eyebrow arch should be from the outer circle to the:
    a. corner of the eyes
    b. iris of the eye upward
    c. outer corner of the nose
    d. inner corner of the eye upward

    ____

CHAPTER 24—NAIL DISEASES AND DISORDERS

1. A normal healthy nail is firm and flexible and should be
   a. smooth and unspotted
   b. uneven and unspotted
   c. unspotted and long
   d. medium length and unspotted ____

2. A nail disorder is classified as a condition that is caused by:
   a. injury or disease
   b. free edge
   c. nail surface
   d. improper care or white spots ____

3. If a client has skin that is infected, inflamed, or swollen, the client should be referred to:
   a. a series of nail treatments
   b. a physician
   c. a licensed manicurist
   d. an upscale salon ____

4. A condition of the nails in which blood clots form under the nail plate is:
   a. damaged nails
   b. swollen nails
   c. bruised nails
   d. eggshell nails ____

5. When performing nail services on a client with nail ridges running vertically down the nail plate, it is recommended that the technician:
   a. carefully remove the nail plate
   b. carefully buff the nail plate
   c. refuse to service the client
   d. refer the client to a medical doctor ____

6. A common nail condition where living skin around the nail splits due to dryness of the skin is:
   a. beau's lines
   b. leukonychia spots
   c. onych
   d. hangnails ____

7. A localized area of increased pigment cells within the matrix bed is responsible for the nail condition:
   a. beau's lines
   b. agnail
   c. melanonychia
   d. melanin ____

8. A common term used to describe a nail with a highly curved nail plate is:
   a. bitten nail
   b. split nail
   c. bruised nail
   d. plicatured nail ____

9. An abnormal nail condition that is the result of damage to the eponychium or hyponychium and occurs when skin is stretched by the nail plate is:
   a. nail pterygium
   b. curved nails
   c. pincer nail
   d. nail cuticle ____

10. Parasites that under some conditions may cause infection to the feet and hands are:
   a. fungi
   b. pusd.
   c. pincer
   mold ____

11. Nail fungi are of concern to the salon because they can be transmitted through unsanitary implements and are:
   a. unhealthy
   b. fragile
   c. contagious
   d. viruses ____

12. A term that should not be used when referring to infections of the fingernails or toenails is:
   a. tinea
   b. bacteria
   c. mold
   d. pathogens ____

13. To prevent fungal organisms on the nail, in addition to the sanitation and disinfection of implements, the technician must properly:
   a. clean and prepare the natural nail plate
   b. clean and prepare the nail cuticle area
   c. remove nail polish remover from nails
   d. file nails with a disposable file ____

14. A typical bacterial infection on the nail plate can be identified in the early stages as a:
   a. blue-black spot under the nail
   b. yellow-green spot on the nail
   c. white spot on the nail bed
   d. black spots on the nail plate ____

15. To avoid the spread of any nail diseases or bacterial infections, it is imperative that the technician use:
   a. strict sanitation and disinfection practices
   b. familiar sanitation practices
   c. strict disinfection and proficient skill techniques
   d. low-level sanitation and disinfection practices ____

16. The lifting of the nail plate from the bed without shedding is a nail disease called:
   a. onycholysis
   b. onychomadesis
   c. nail psoriasis
   d. ingrown nails ____

17. A bacterial inflammation surrounding the nail tissue that may be the result of excessive exposure to water is:
    a. paronychia
    b. tinea pedis
    c. salmon patches
    d. pyogenic ____

18. The medical term for fungal infections associated with the feet is:
    a. tinea pathogenic
    b. tinea pedis
    c. tinea alopecia
    d. paronychia ____

19. The technical term used to describe bitten nails is:
    a. onychophagy
    b. onychorrhexis
    c. onycholysis
    d. onyx ____

20. The naturally occurring skin bacteria that can grow out of control and cause an infection if conditions are correct is:
    a. melanonychia
    b. pseudomonas aeruginosa
    c. leukonychia
    d. pterygium ____

CHAPTER 25—MANICURING

1. A manicuring table lamp should have an incandescent bulb with wattage no higher than:
   a. 10 to 30 watts
   b. 40 to 60 watts
   c. 70 to 90 watts
   d. 100 to 120 watts ____

2. Disinfection containers for manicure implements should be large enough for implements to be:
   a. partially immersed
   b. removed with hands
   c. completely immersed
   d. completely cleaned ____

3. Lids are required on disinfectant containers to prevent:
   a. spilling
   b. contamination
   c. immersion
   d. sharing ____

4. Manicuring implements should be placed in the disinfectant container after being:
   a. used several times
   b. used by the client
   c. properly marked
   d. properly cleaned ____

5. A wooden pusher used to remove cuticle tissue is disposable and should be:
   a. sanitized and reused
   b. discarded after each use
   c. placed in a cabinet drawer
   d. washed with soap and water ____

6. A metal pusher is used to push back the eponychium and gently scrape cuticle tissue from the:
   a. natural nail root
   b. natural nail plate
   c. nail free edge
   d. nail matrix ____

7. Fine grit abrasives are designed for removing very fine scratches and:
   a. buffing and polishing
   b. aggressive buffing
   c. beveling the nail
   d. reducing nail length ____

8. To bevel a nail, use gentle pressure and angle the file with a:
   a. 60-degree angle
   b. 90-degree angle
   c. 45-degree angle
   d. straight angle ____

9. Clean abrasives or implements stored in plastic bags or sealed airtight containers promote:
   a. air circulation
   b. bacterial growth
   c. storage problems
   d. ineffective storage ____

10. A nipper should be used to carefully trim away the:
    a. nail plate
    b. nail free edge
    c. cuticle area
    d. tags of dead skin ____

11. A buffer that shines the nail plate without the use of dry buffing powder is a(n):
    a. abrasive buffer
    b. wooden pusher
    c. three-way buffer
    d. electric dryer ____

12. A tool used to shorten the length of the natural nail plate is a(n):
    a. electric dryer
    b. wooden pusher
    c. nail clipper
    d. nail nipper ____

13. The time necessary to properly clean and disinfect implements after each use is:
    a. 10 minutes
    b. 20 minutes
    c. 60 minutes
    d. 30 minutes ____

14. Brushes used in products that do not harbor the growth of pathogens are considered:
    a. renewable brushes
    b. self-disinfecting
    c. bacteria free
    d. self-cleaning ____

15. Small fiber-free squares used to apply or remove product are:
    a. cotton
    b. linen
    c. fibers
    d. pledgets ____

16. Nail products should be removed from their containers using a:
    a. plastic or metal spatula
    b. finger
    c. plastic or metal brush
    d. cotton ____

17. Cosmetic products containing a high water content provide the growth opportunity for:
    a. pathogens
    b. containers
    c. fibers
    d. vapors ____

18. The use of bar soap is not recommended as it may:
    a. be expensive
    b. be inexpensive
    c. harbor bacteria
    d. spread ethyl ____

19. When removing nail polish from wrap-type nail enhancements, use a solvent that is:
    a. acetone
    b. non-acetone
    c. quick
    d. conditioning ____

20. Removers that are used to dissolve and remove polish contain solvents of ethyl acetate or:
    a. mineral oil
    b. sodium
    c. acetone
    d. potassium ____

21. A product designed to loosen and dissolve dead tissue from the nail plate is:
    a. moisturizing lotion
    b. nonacetone remover
    c. polish remover
    d. cuticle remover ____

22. A product designed to improve adhesion of polish to the natural nail is a:
    a. top coat
    b. nail hardener
    c. reinforcing coat
    d. base coat ____

23. Nail hardeners that cause adverse reactions to skin may contain:
    a. formaldehyde
    b. resins
    c. acrylic
    d. dimethyl urea ____

24. Product information including safe handling, first aid, and proper storage is required in:
    a. Manufacturers Direction Sheets
    b. Material Supply Order Forms
    c. Material Safety Data Sheets
    d. Material Disposal Sheets ____

25. Generally, it is recommended that the shape of the nail plate enhances the overall:
    a. shape of the cuticle
    b. shape of the fingertip
    c. length of the nail
    d. shape of the hands ____

26. The five basic nail shapes are:
    a. square, pointed, oval, flat, and slender
    c. square, squoval, round, pointed, and oval
    b. slender, oval, squoval, square, and pointed
    d. pointed, square, narrow, round, and strong ____

27. Should a client be accidentally cut and blood drawn, the first precautionary step is to:
    a. put on gloves and inform client
    b. clean with antiseptic solution
    c. stanch bleeding with pressure
    d. discard used materials ____

28. The three individual procedures for a basic manicure should include:
    a. pre-service, post-service, and disinfection procedures
    b. pre-service, actual service, and post-service
    c. consultation, pre-service, and service performed
    d. pre-service, post-service, and recommendations ____

29. Success in nail polish application is achieved by using four coats including:
    a. one base coat, one polish color, and two top coats
    b. two polish color, one top coat, and one sealer coat
    c. one base coat, two polish color, and one top coat
    d. one base coat, one polish color, and two top coats ____

30. Massage manipulations should be executed using:
    a. fast rubbing movements
    b. rhythmic and smooth movements
    c. fast, pulsating movements
    d. fast, rotating movements ____

31. The massage movement where the technician holds the client's wrist and bends it back and forth slowly is a form of:
    a. joint movement
    b. circular movement
    c. rotating movement
    d. palm effleurage ____

32. Vigorous joint massage should not be performed if a client has a joint injury or:
    a. arthritis
    b. psoriasis
    c. migraines
    d. artificial nails ____

33. Sitting or working in uncomfortable, strained positions can lead to back, neck, or shoulder injuries and result in:
    a. temporary trauma
    b. carpal tunnel trauma disorders
    c. temporary relaxation
    d. cumulative trauma ____

34. Spa manicures encompass extensive knowledge of nail care and:
    a. skin care treatments
    b. consultations
    c. towel applications
    d. lotion applications ____

35. Spa manicures include massage and skin exfoliation for polishing, smoothing, and enhancing:
    a. massage ambiance
    b. oily cosmetics
    c. professional product penetration
    d. client's preference for cosmetics ____

CHAPTER 26—PEDICURING

1. Pedicure procedures include trimming, shaping, and polishing toenails; exfoliating skin; and:
   a. foot masques
   b. foot massage services
   c. nail plate dissolvers
   d. recommending hair ____

2. To ensure healthy, happy feet, professional pedicure services should be performed:
   a. yearly
   b. weekly
   c. monthly
   d. daily ____

3. A pedicure tool used to exfoliate dry skin or smooth calluses is a:
   a. rasp
   b. paddle
   c. curette
   d. clipper ____

4. A pedicuring station should include a comfortable chair for the client, a footrest for the client, and a(n):
   a. designer chair for the nail professional
   b. designed stool for the client
   c. ergonomic stool for the nail professional
   d. ergonomic chair for the nail professional ____

5. To be effective in a pedicure bath, liquid soaps should contain a(n):
   a. scented oil
   b. antibacterial soap
   c. mild detergent
   d. strong detergent ____

6. Lotions, oils, and creams are used to condition and moisturize feet and for:
   a. performing a foot massage
   b. disinfecting the foot spa
   c. applying polish to the toenails
   d. removing polish from the toenails ____

7. A metal file that is designed to be used in a specific fashion is a:
   a. board
   b. brush
   c. curette
   d. rasp ____

8. The tool used to exfoliate dry skin or smooth calluses during a pedicure service is a:
   a. foot bath
   b. foot file
   c. pedicure clipper
   d. toe separator ____

9. When working on the foot, it should be grasped between the thumb and fingers at the:
   a. bottom of the foot
   b. heel area
   c. mid-tarsal area
   d. ankle area ____

10. The actual pedicure procedure has five basic steps: the soak, nail care, skin care,
   a. polish, and rebook
   b. massage, and polish
   c. massage, and waxing
   d. polish, and exfoliating ____

11. When performing a pedicure, apply a firm grip on the client's foot to:
   a. produce a tickling sensation
   b. calm the client
   c. waste finger motions
   d. lock the ankle area ____

12. When clipping toenails, extra care should be exercised to avoid breaking the:
   a. hyponychium
   b. dermis
   c. pressure point
   d. elastin ____

13. To properly disinfect a foot spa after each pedicure service, the nail technician is required to perform the following steps:
   a. Drain and remove water and contaminants, add more soap and water, and use.
   b. Drain and remove water and contaminants, clean surface, disinfect with approved disinfectant, rinse, and dry.
   c. Drain and remove water, disinfect with approved disinfectant, rinse, and dry.
   d. Change water, add soap , disinfect with approved disinfectant, thoroughly rinse, and dry. ____

14. The procedure for cleaning a foot spa at the end of the day is: remove and clean screen of trapped debris, wash screen and inlet and totally immerse in approved disinfectant, then:
   a. flush system with warm water for 5 minutes, rinse, and air dry
   b. rinse out system with warm water for 2 minutes, rinse with cold water, and dry with sponge
   c. flush system with low-sudsing soap and water for 10 minutes, rinse, drain, and air-dry
   d. rinse system with low-sudsing soap and water for 5 minutes, rinse, drain, and towel dry ____

15. The weekly maintenance procedure for foot spas requires the disinfectant solution to remain in the foot spa at least:
   a. 4 to 5 hours
   b. 6 to 10 hours
   c. 1 or 2 hours
   d. 2 to 3 hours ____

16. Foot massage performed correctly is relaxing to the client, is therapeutic, and:
    a. stimulates nail growth
    b. increases foot pressure
    c. stimulates muscle growth
    d. stimulates blood flow ____

17. The massage movement used to stretch the muscles and tendons is:
    a. petrissage
    b. effleurage
    c. tapping
    d. kneading ____

18. A product that should never be placed in the foot bath with the client's feet is a:
    a. solution
    b. antiseptic
    c. magnesium salt
    d. disinfectant ____

19. Creams or lotions used to help in the removal and smoothing of dry, flaky skin and calluses are:
    a. massage preparations
    b. natural oils
    c. abrasive scrubs
    d. moisturized agents ____

20. Alkaline cuticle removers should never be applied to:
    a. resins and adhesives
    b. living skin
    c. massage oil products
    d. nail polish ____

21. Professional strength callus softener products usually contain sodium hydroxide or:
    a. lactic acid
    b. sodium chloride
    c. hydrogen peroxide
    d. mineral clays ____

22. A hot paraffin bath should not be provided to a client with:
    a. seasonal allergies
    b. diabetic-related problems
    c. vitamin deficiency
    d. premature aging ____

23. A small "ice cream scooper"-shaped implement used for efficient removal of debris from nail folds and cuticle area is a:
    a. nipper
    b. clipper
    c. curette
    d. spatula ____

24. Toenail clippers used for a pedicure service should have:
    a. double edges
    b. fairly fine points
    c. fairly straight edges
    d. two even edges ____

25. Nail rasps are a tool specifically designed to file:
    a. in several directions
    b. across nail grooves
    c. along edges
    d. in one direction ____

CHAPTER 27—NAIL TIPS, WRAPS, AND NO-LIGHT GELS

1. Plastic, premolded forms adhered to natural nails to add length or support nail enhancement products are:
   a. nail wraps
   b. nail tips
   c. nail overlays
   d. nail adhesives ____

2. Nail tips break easily without the reinforcement called a(n):
   a. overlay
   b. adhesive
   c. full-well
   d. activator ____

3. A rough surface tool used to shape, smooth, and remove the surface shine on a nail is a(n):
   a. emery board
   b. shine remover
   c. gel activator
   d. abrasive board ____

4. The term used to describe the thickness of nail adhesives is:
   a. strength
   b. viscosity
   c. durability
   d. safety ____

5. Nail tips should never cover more than:
   a. one-half of the nail plate
   b. all the nail plate
   c. one-third of the natural nail plate
   d. tip of natural nail ____

6. The shallow depression area of a nail tip is the:
   a. well
   b. contact
   c. applicator
   d. gelled ____

7. When placing nail tips on the natural nail plate, the technique used is:
   a. stop, hold, and release
   b. stop, rock, and hold
   c. rock, hold, and free
   d. rock, slide, and release ____

8. When blending a nail tip at the contact area, the fine-grit buff block should be held:
   a. at a 45-degree angle against the nail plate
   b. at a right angle against the nail plate
   c. deep into the nail plate
   d. flat across the surface of the nail plate ____

9. The action used with a wooden pusher to remove softened nail tips is:
   a. pull gently with pusher
   b. slide off with clippers
   c. slide off with pusher
   d. nip off with nippers ____

10. Nail enhancements using nail-size pieces of cloth or paper bonded to the nail plate are:
    a. nail wraps
    b. gel nails
    c. adhesive wraps
    d. opaque wraps ____

11. The strongest material used as a nail wrap is:
    a. silk
    b. paper
    c. fiberglass
    d. linen ____

12. A product that accelerates the curing process of resins and adhesives is a(n):
    a. heat spike
    b. extender tip
    c. activator
    d. plastic strip ____

13. A product applied to the surface of natural nails to remove moisture and improve adhesion is a:
    a. nail blender
    b. nail activator
    c. nail adhesive
    d. nail dehydrator ____

14. When applying nail wraps, to prevent the transfer of oil and debris from the technician to the client, use:
    a. gloves
    b. flexible plastic sheets
    c. wooden spatulas
    d. small pieces of cotton ____

15. Nail wraps should be rebalanced with resin and new fabric after:
    a. 6 weeks
    b. 8 weeks
    c. 4 weeks
    d. 2 months ____

16. A fabric piece cut to completely cover a crack or break in a nail wrap is a:
    a. stress strip
    b. repair patch
    c. rebalance batch
    d. refill strip ____

17. A gel-like material that requires an activator to cure is:
    a. gel light application
    b. no-cure gel application
    c. resin gel application
    d. no-light gel application ____

18. The improper use of activators can cause a heat spike to the client and:
    a. polymer damage
    b. pulling sensation
    c. surface shine
    d. nail bed damage ____

19. To avoid damaging nail wraps when removing existing polish, use a(n):
    a. acetone remover
    b. oil accelerator
    c. resin softener
    d. nonacetone remover ____

20. An implement similar to a nail clipper, designed especially for use on nail tips, is a:
    a. tip nipper
    b. tip cutter
    c. stress cutter
    d. tip buffer ____

CHAPTER 28—ACRYLIC (METHACRYLATE) NAILS

1. Acrylic (methacrylate) nail enhancements are created by combining monomer liquid with:
   a. monomer powder
   b. polymer powder
   c. liquid powder
   d. molecular powder ____

2. Nail enhancements sculptured with the use of polymer powder are called:
   a. monomer nails
   b. protective nails
   c. synthetic nails
   d. acrylic nails ____

3. Brushes recommended for the application of acrylic (methacrylate) product are:
   a. natural hair
   b. nylon bristles
   c. mixed hair
   d. plastic bristles ____

4. When applying product, the brush is immersed into monomer and the tip of the brush is:
   a. dragged across the surface of the dry polymer powder
   b. pushed gently into the dry polymer powder
   c. immersed into the dry polymer powder
   d. touched to the surface of the dry polymer powder ____

5. As monomer liquid absorbs a polymer powder, the product formed at the tip of the brush is referred to as a:
   a. monomer bead
   b. bead of product
   c. chemical reaction
   d. molded product ____

6. Polymer powder is made using a special chemical reaction called:
   a. polychain
   b. monomer chains
   c. polymerization
   d. methacrylate chains ____

7. In the process of creating acrylic (methacrylate) nails, trillions of monomers are linked together to create:
   a. additives
   b. long chains
   c. dry chemicals
   d. long absorptions ____

8. Additives are responsible for the product durability and color stability of the product, and they ensure:
   a. complete cure or set
   b. complete beads
   c. proper procedure
   d. proper disposal ____

9. Additives used to control the set or curing time in monomer liquids are called:
   a. accelerators and adhesives
   b. controllers and resins
   c. catalysts and initiators
   d. adhesives and catalysts ____

10. Initiators in polymer powder cause monomer molecules to permanently link together and form:
    a. short monomer chains
    b. long polymer chains
    c. long polymer forms
    d. short chain reactions ____

11. The initiator added to polymer powder is:
    a. hydrogen peroxide
    b. catalyst peroxide
    c. sodium hydroxide
    d. benzoyl peroxide ____

12. To ensure the proper curing when using nail enhancement products:
    a. use a variety of products
    b. intermix products as necessary
    c. mix manufacturer product lines
    d. do not mix manufacturer product lines ____

13. Acrylic (methacrylate) overlays and nail enhancements can be created using one color powder if the client wears:
    a. clear polish all the time
    b. nail polish all the time
    c. semiliquid nail polish
    d. natural colors all the time ____

14. The amount of monomer liquid and polymer powder used to create a bead is called the:
    a. dry bead
    b. liquid bead
    c. powder ratio
    d. mix ratio ____

15. If the consistency of a bead contains too little powder, the enhancement may not:
    a. file easily
    b. balance easily
    c. cure correctly
    d. polish easily ____

16. Surface moisture and oil on the natural nail plate can be removed with nail antiseptic or:
    a. nail dehydrators
    b. corrosive agents
    c. heavy primers
    d. nail hydrators ____

17. The use of acid-based nail primers may result in:
    a. skin burns or injury
    b. lifting of skin
    c. skin rejuvenation
    d. better adhesion ____

18. Acrylic (methacrylate) nail enhancements reach their ultimate strength in:
    a. 24 to 48 hours
    b. 5 to 10 hours
    c. 30 to 45 minutes
    d. 12 to 15 hours ____

19. Nail adhesives used to secure nail tips to natural nails are all based on:
    a. catalyst monomers
    b. cyanoacrylate polymers
    c. acetone inhibitors
    d. cyanoacrylate monomers ____

20. To prevent product contamination, a dappen dish should have:
    a. a loosely fitted lid
    b. a tightly fitted lid
    c. a large opening
    d. an evaporation lid ____

21. The shelf life of nail adhesives can be as short as:
    a. 1 year
    b. 8 months
    c. 6 months
    d. 2 years ____

22. Unused monomer poured back into the original container will cause product:
    a. spilling
    b. sensitivity
    c. customizing
    d. contamination ____

23. The type of glove recommended for nail salon services is:
    a. nylon polymer
    b. hard plastic
    c. latex polymer
    d. nitrile polymer ____

24. The area that should not be cut when applying multiuse nail forms is the:
    a. nail fold
    b. hyponychium
    c. cuticle fold
    d. nail root ____

25. The bead of product for shaping the free edge should have a:
    a. wet consistency
    b. balanced consistency
    c. medium consistency
    d. large consistency ____

26. The time required for a product to properly clean brushes is determined by:
    a. the technician
    b. the client
    c. the manufacturer's directions
    d. necessity ____

27. When placing the second ball of acrylic on the free edge, use a medium consistency and place on the nail plate below the first bead and:
    a. next to the side wall edge line and on the right side of the nail
    b. next to the free edge line within 1/8 inch of the nail
    c. next to the free edge line in the center of the nail
    d. on the nail plate within 1/8 inch of the cuticle area ____

28. For natural looking nails, the product application must be smooth and thin at the:
    a. eponychium, free edge, and base
    b. free edge and side walls
    c. side walls, free edge, and eponychium
    d. side walls, base, and free edge ____

29. In rebalancing acrylic (methacrylate) nail enhancements, the nail is thinned down and reduced in thickness and:
    a. the nail will be reduced in width
    b. the apex of the nail will be removed
    c. the nail will be filed
    d. the nail will be refinished

    ____

30. The area between the existing acrylic product and new growth of the nail plate is the:
    a. thinned area
    b. balance area
    c. nail unit
    d. ledge

    ____

CHAPTER 29—UV GELS

1. The ingredients used in UV gels are from a subfamily of acrylics called:
   a. monomers
   b. acrylates
   c. enhancements
   d. polymers ____

2. Recently developed UV gel technologies utilize chemistry from:
   a. monoacrylics
   b. polyacrylates
   c. methacrylates
   d. monomer powders ____

3. A short chain of monomers not long enough to be considered a polymer is a(n):
   a. additive
   b. adhesive
   c. oligomer
   d. resin ____

4. Newer UV gel systems use chemicals called:
   a. monomers
   b. urethane methacrylates
   c. adhesive based
   d. resin based ____

5. An advantage of UV gel systems is:
   a. color
   b. durability
   c. liquid polymer
   d. low odor ____

6. The UV gel application process differs from other types of nail enhancements; with a UV gel procedure:
   a. each layer of product is a different color when exposed to UV light
   b. each layer of product must cure or harden with exposure to UV light
   c. product is applied without the use of any UV light
   d. product must dry between layers with white lights ____

7. UV gel products are usually packaged in opaque pots or:
   a. dark bottles
   b. individual applications
   c. large tubes
   d. squeeze tubes ____

8. A measure of how much electricity a bulb consumes is:
   a. voltage
   b. amps
   c. wattage
   d. power ____

9. Brushes used in the application of UV gels are:
   a. human
   b. synthetic
   c. sable
   d. long ____

10. To improve the shelf life of nail adhesives, store them at room temperature between:
    a. 20°F and 40°F
    b. 45°F and 55°F
    c. 60°F and 85°F
    d. 90°F and 100°F ____

11. Nail tips applied with a UV gel procedure should be shortened and filed prior to the gel application to prevent:
    a. the client from spending extra time in the salon
    b. the gel seal from being broken during the filing procedure
    c. the gel application from curing correctly during the filing procedure
    d. skin irritations ____

12. The time required to cure each layer of a UV gel product is determined by:
    a. manufacturer's instructions
    b. the length of the nail
    c. the client
    d. the number of coats applied ____

13. UV gels cure with a tacky surface called a(n):
    a. second layer
    b. contour layer
    c. inhibition layer
    d. primary layer ____

14. The final layer of UV gel should be brushed under the free edge of the natural nail enhancement to create a(n):
    a. ledge
    b. seal
    c. angle
    d. adhesion ____

15. First UV gel is called the:
    a. base coat gel
    b. finishing gel
    c. sealing gel
    d. building gel ____

16. To reduce client skin irritation and sensitivity when applying the base coat gel:
    a. pull the UV gel quickly across the nail plate
    b. leave a tiny free margin between the UV gel and the skin
    c. remove the inhibition layer
    d. press hard with the brush ____

17. The oily shine on natural nails should be removed using:
    a. round circles
    b. vertical strokes
    c. round strokes
    d. firm pressure ____

18. UV gel enhancements must be rebalanced every:
    a. 2 to 3 weeks
    b. 4 to 5 weeks
    c. 5 to 6 weeks
    d. 6 to 8 weeks ____

19. The abrasive used to check and refine the nail contour for UV gel nails is:
    a. nonabrasive
    b. fine abrasive
    c. medium abrasive
    d. harsh abrasive ____

20. Third UV gel is called the finisher or:
    a. builder gel
    b. sealer gel
    c. building gel
    d. adhesion gel ____

CHAPTER 30—SEEKING EMPLOYMENT

1. Most professionals have become successful through self-motivation, energy, and:
   a. technical skills
   b. persistence
   c. talent
   d. opportunity ____

2. Of all the factors that affect licensing test performance, the most important is mastery of:
   a. technical skills
   b. organizing handouts
   c. course content
   d. school notes ____

3. When taking a licensure test, even if you have truly learned the material, it is still very beneficial to have:
   a. a well-organized notebook
   b. a detailed vocabulary list
   c. listening skills
   d. strong test-taking skills ____

4. The process of reaching logical conclusions by employing logical reasoning is:
   a. studying the night before the exam
   b. cramming the night before the exam
   c. marking skipped questions
   d. deductive reasoning ____

5. When reaffirming a goal by reviewing a number of important questions, it is recommended to perform a(n):
   a. personal inventory of characteristics and skills
   b. complete Inventory of practical skills
   c. inventory of personal likes and qualities
   d. personal inventory of knowledge and skills ____

6. A salon owned by an individual or two or more partners with 3 to 40 styling stations is classified as a:
   a. full-service salon
   b. small independent salon
   c. independent salon chain
   d. neighborhood salon ____

7. Independent salon chains are basic or full-service salons and day spas consisting of five or more salons that are owned by:
   a. five or more partners
   b. large corporations
   c. one individual
   d. one individual or two or more partners ____

8. A form of chain salons that share a national name, consistent image, and business formula throughout are:
   a. franchise salons
   b. large chains
   c. privately owned
   d. business salons ____

9. A salon business that offers higher-priced services with luxurious extras is a:
   a. budget salon or day spa
   b. booth rental establishment
   c. basic value-priced operation
   d. high-end image salon or day spa ____

10. A written summary provided to employers of your education and work experience is a:
   a. job application
   b. résumé
   c. cover letter
   d. personal inventory ____

11. Skills mastered at other jobs that can be put to use in another position are called:
   a. transferable skills
   b. accomplishment skills
   c. salary references
   d. training skills ____

12. A bound collection of photos and documents used to showcase your skills and accomplishments is a(n):
   a. portfolio
   b. assessment
   c. resume
   d. summary ____

13. A technique of making contact with salons and professionals is called:
   a. gathering
   b. establishing
   c. advertising
   d. networking ____

14. After doing a salon site visit, it is important to send the salon representative a:
   a. résumé
   b. cover letter
   c. thank-you note
   d. declining note ____

15. When selecting and interviewing salons for potential employment opportunities, it is important that the stylist make:
   a. informed comparisons
   b. hasty choices
   c. no comparisons
   d. inappropriate remarks ____

16. After observing and targeting salons for employment opportunities, the next step would be to contact the establishments by:
   a. visiting the salon when they are busy
   b. sending a résumé and cover letter
   c. contacting the salon manger by phone
   d. completing a job application ____

17. When preparing for an interview, necessary employment information and materials include:
    a. identification and social security number
    b. drivers license and high school diploma
    c. social security number and cell phone number
    d. contact numbers and school certificate of completion ____

18. Issues and questions that cannot be included in an employment application or interview include:
    a. date of birth if applicant is younger than 18
    b. race, religion, date of birth, and national origin
    c. medical conditions and salary
    d. citizenship, drugs, and smoking ____

19. When you take pride in your work and commit yourself to doing a good job for your clients and employer, you have a strong:
    a. work ethic
    b. position statement
    c. employment advantage
    d. technical skill ____

20. On the day of a salon interview, a warm, friendly smile and confident posture will project a(n):
    a. good interview
    b. achievement
    c. false impression
    d. positive first impression ____

CHAPTER 31—ON THE JOB

1. Compared to cosmetology school, you will find that your real-world work schedule will be:
   a. more flexible
   b. less flexible
   c. equally flexible
   d. not at all flexible ____

2. When seeking employment, it is important to be honest with yourself as you evaluate your skills to determine:
   a. how great your skills are
   b. the many services you are proficient at performing
   c. the type of position that is right for you
   d. the money that you can charge ____

3. The number one thing to remember in a service business is that your work revolves around:
   a. serving your clients
   b. how well you feel
   c. the time of day
   d. how many hours you work ____

4. To be a good team player requires that you practice and perfect your:
   a. telephone skills
   b. personal life
   c. people skills
   d. scheduled shifts ____

5. The document that outlines all the duties and responsibilities of a particular position is a:
   a. duty list
   b. job description
   c. daily chores summary
   d. job document ____

6. When you accept a job offer, what you actually get paid for your work is called:
   a. check
   b. cash
   c. incentives
   d. compensation ____

7. In most salons the three standard methods of employee compensation are:
   a. salary, commission, and retail sales
   b. commission, salary plus commission, and employee incentives
   c. salary, commission, and salary plus commission
   d. check, commission, salary, and bonuses ____

8. An excellent job opportunity for a new cosmetology school graduate is as a(n):
   a. assistant
   b. platform artist
   c. practitioner
   d. receptionist ____

9. For the beginning salon professional without a clientele, the best compensation method would be:
   a. weekly
   b. commission only
   c. with no taxes
   d. a salary ____

10. Compensation paid to an employee as a direct result of the total amount of service dollars generated for the salon is:
   a. commission
   b. gratuities
   c. clientele
   d. salary ____

11. A compensation structure that is used to motivate and increase practitioner productivity is:
   a. tax-free salaries
   b. salary plus commission
   c. commission only
   d. regular compensation ____

12. Income provided in acknowledgment of satisfactory service that must be reported on one's income tax return is:
   a. tips
   b. taxes
   c. retail sales
   d. referrals ____

13. Employer and coworker feedback on technical abilities, career direction, and growth should be provided during a(n):
   a. client service
   b. referral program
   c. employee evaluation
   d. employee lunch break ____

14. To manage expenses and debts, financial planning includes a:
   a. mathematical genius
   b. personal budget
   c. personal diary
   d. free spending log ____

15. The practice of recommending and selling additional professional services to clients is:
   a. retail sales
   b. upselling services
   c. part of the duties and responsibilities
   d. part of the job description ____

16. Recommending and selling professional products to clients for at-home care is:
   a. economics
   b. commission
   c. advertising
   d. retailing ____

17. To be successful in sales, the practitioner must be ambitious and determined and have:
   a. a good client
   b. an assertive personality
   c. a good personality
   d. a personal preference ____

18. In the psychology of selling, it is the job of the practitioner to figure out the reason a person may want to buy a product and determine the client's:
    a. intelligence
    b. motives for buying salon products
    c. financial situation
    d. stress level

    ____

19. Clients whom you service on a regular basis are referred to as your:
    a. reliable clients
    b. good clients
    c. complaining clients
    d. client base

    ____

20. The process of scheduling clients for return visits to the salon is referred to as:
    a. selling
    b. suggestions
    c. rebooking
    d. referrals

    ____

CHAPTER 32—THE SALON BUSINESS

1. Being a successful businessperson requires experience, a genuine love of people, and solid:
   a. technical skills
   b. management skills
   c. business licenses
   d. insurance policies ____

2. Where allowed by state law, a desirable alternative salon ownership is the practice of:
   a. booth rental
   b. booth sales
   c. leased space
   d. unlicensed activity ____

3. When opening a salon, two of the most important factors in predicting the success of the business are:
   a. location and services
   b. visibility and products
   c. visibility and accessibility
   d. competition and products ____

4. When obtaining financing to open a business, it is essential to develop a(n):
   a. employee handbook
   b. business plan
   c. tax shelter
   d. service menu ____

5. The professional trained in the gathering of accurate financial information needed in developing a business plan is a(n):
   a. relative
   b. coworker
   c. vendor
   d. accountant ____

6. Purchasing the insurance required for operating a salon is the responsibility of the:
   a. salon owner
   b. building owner
   c. salon employee
   d. salon supplier ____

7. Another name for an individual owner with complete control of a business is:
   a. leader
   b. manager
   c. sole proprietor
   d. receptionist ____

8. In a partnership, two or more people share ownership, although the ownership shares may not always be:
   a. fair
   b. friendly
   c. equal
   d. operational ____

9. Incorporating is one of the best ways for a business owner to protect:
   a. personal assets
   b. unmanageable debts
   c. personal secrets
   d. supply inventory ____

10. A business advantage of a corporation when raising capital (money) is that a corporation may issue shares or:
    a. tax shelters
    b. stock certificates
    c. liability insurance
    d. business charters ____

11. To avoid any misunderstandings between contracting parties in the purchase a salon, the details of the sale should be written in the:
    a. building lease agreement
    b. business plan
    c. purchase and sales agreement
    d. professional name ____

12. Business records that are used to record all income are classified as:
    a. receipts
    b. invoices
    c. expenses
    d. retail ____

13. Records that help maintain an overstocking or shortage of supplies and are used to establish the net worth of a business are:
    a. invoice and revenue records
    b. purchase and inventory records
    c. sales and employee records
    d. expense and payroll records ____

14. Supplies used in the daily business operation are considered:
    a. retail supplies
    b. consumer supplies
    c. consumption supplies
    d. inventory supplies ____

15. Supplies purchased by a salon with the intention of selling these products to clients are:
    a. retail supplies
    b. consumption supplies
    c. special supplies
    d. client supplies ____

16. When planning and constructing the best physical layout for a salon, the primary concern should be:
    a. color scheme
    b. salon furniture
    c. salon carpeting
    d. maximum efficiency ____

17. To employees, a top priority for salon owners should be to always meet:
    a. employee evaluations
    b. incentives
    c. payroll obligations
    d. preferences ____

18. One of the most important duties of the receptionist is:
    a. booking appointments
    b. making reservations
    c. personal calls
    d. filing ____

19. The best form of advertising for a salon is a(n):
    a. radio spot
    b. newspaper
    c. unhappy client
    d. satisfied client

    ____

20. An important aspect of a salon's financial success revolves around the sale of:
    a. gift certificates
    b. additional salon services
    c. key chains
    d. direct mail

    ____

Part II: Answers to Exam Review for Cosmetology

CHAPTER 1—HISTORY AND CAREER OPPORTUNITIES

1. b	6. a	11. a
2. d	7. c	12. c
3. b	8. b	13. a
4. c	9. a	14. c
5. d	10. b	15. c

CHAPTER 2—LIFE SKILLS

1. b	6. c
2. c	7. c
3. a	8. a
4. c	9. d
5. b	10. a

CHAPTER 3—YOUR PROFESSIONAL IMAGE

1. d	6. b
2. a	7. a
3. d	8. a
4. a	9. a
5. d	10. c

CHAPTER 4—COMMUNICATING FOR SUCCESS

1. d	6. b	11. c
2. b	7. a	12. a
3. a	8. b	13. b
4. d	9. b	14. b
5. a	10. a	15. a

CHAPTER 5—INFECTION CONTROL: PRINCIPLES AND PRACTICES

1. c	11. d	21. a	31. a	41. a
2. b	12. a	22. b	32. b	42. b
3. a	13. c	23. c	33. a	43. c
4. b	14. a	24. b	34. d	44. a
5. b	15. a	25. d	35. a	45. a
6. d	16. b	26. a	36. b	46. a
7. c	17. a	27. b	37. c	47. a
8. c	18. b	28. c	38. a	48. b
9. d	19. c	29. d	39. b	49. a
10. a	20. a	30. c	40. d	50. c

CHAPTER 5—INFECTION CONTROL: PRINCIPLES AND PRACTICES (*continued*)

51. a	56. a	61. a	66. c	71. d
52. b	57. d	62. d	67. c	72. b
53. c	58. b	63. a	68. a	73. a
54. a	59. a	64. a	69. b	74. b
55. d	60. c	65. b	70. c	75. a

CHAPTER 6—GENERAL ANATOMY AND PHYSIOLOGY

1. a	15. b	29. a	43. d	57. b
2. b	16. b	30. c	44. a	58. c
3. a	17. c	31. d	45. d	59. a
4. d	18. c	32. b	46. b	60. c
5. c	19. b	33. a	47. a	61. b
6. b	20. c	34. c	48. d	62. c
7. c	21. a	35. c	49. b	63. b
8. a	22. d	36. b	50. d	64. c
9. a	23. b	37. a	51. b	65. b
10. d	24. a	38. d	52. b	66. a
11. b	25. b	39. a	53. b	
12. a	26. b	40. b	54. b	
13. c	27. c	41. c	55. c	
14. d	28. d	42. a	56. b	

CHAPTER 7—SKIN STRUCTURE AND GROWTH

1. b	8. a	15. b	22. d	29. d
2. c	9. c	16. c	23. a	30. a
3. b	10. a	17. d	24. c	31. c
4. a	11. b	18. a	25. b	32. b
5. c	12. a	19. c	26. c	33. a
6. d	13. b	20. b	27. d	34. b
7. b	14. a	21. a	28. a	35. d

CHAPTER 8—NAIL STRUCTURE AND GROWTH

1. b	6. a	11. c	16. a	21. d
2. c	7. c	12. a	17. a	22. c
3. b	8. a	13. d	18. b	23. b
4. d	9. b	14. a	19. d	24. a
5. d	10. b	15. c	20. a	25. d

CHAPTER 9—PROPERTIES OF THE HAIR AND SCALP

1. b	5. a	9. c	13. c	17. b
2. c	6. c	10. b	14. a	18. b
3. b	7. b	11. c	15. b	19. b
4. d	8. a	12. c	16. c	20. c

CHAPTER 9—PROPERTIES OF THE HAIR AND SCALP
(*continued*)

21. d	31. b	41. b	51. a	61. c
22. b	32. d	42. c	52. c	62. a
23. c	33. a	43. a	53. d	63. a
24. a	34. a	44. a	54. b	64. b
25. a	35. c	45. c	55. a	65. c
26. d	36. d	46. b	56. b	66. a
27. c	37. a	47. a	57. c	67. a
28. a	38. c	48. b	58. a	68. a
29. d	39. a	49. d	59. d	69. a
30. a	40. a	50. c	60. a	70. b

CHAPTER 10—BASICS OF CHEMISTRY

1. b	8. a	15. a	22. a	29. d
2. c	9. b	16. b	23. b	30. d
3. a	10. b	17. a	24. b	31. b
4. b	11. d	18. c	25. c	32. b
5. c	12. a	19. b	26. a	33. c
6. b	13. c	20. d	27. c	34. a
7. d	14. b	21. c	28. b	35. a

CHAPTER 11—BASICS OF ELECTRICITY

1. a	6. a	11. a	16. d	21. a
2. b	7. b	12. b	17. b	22. a
3. b	8. b	13. a	18. a	23. a
4. a	9. d	14. c	19. c	24. a
5. d	10. c	15. a	20. c	25. a

CHAPTER 12—PRINCIPLES OF HAIR DESIGN

1. b	7. d	13. b	19. b	25. a
2. a	8. a	14. d	20. a	26. d
3. c	9. b	15. a	21. d	27. c
4. a	10. a	16. a	22. a	28. d
5. c	11. d	17. c	23. c	29. a
6. d	12. a	18. a	24. a	30. b

CHAPTER 13—SHAMPOOING, RINSING, AND CONDITIONING

1. a	8. a	15. a	22. c	29. c
2. c	9. c	16. c	23. c	30. a
3. b	10. a	17. a	24. b	31. b
4. c	11. d	18. d	25. b	32. c
5. d	12. b	19. a	26. d	33. a
6. b	13. b	20. b	27. a	34. d
7. c	14. d	21. a	28. a	35. b

CHAPTER 14—HAIRCUTTING

1. b	14. a	27. c	40. c	53. c
2. c	15. d	28. d	41. a	54. d
3. b	16. b	29. b	42. b	55. b
4. d	17. c	30. b	43. d	56. a
5. a	18. c	31. c	44. b	57. b
6. b	19. c	32. a	45. a	58. c
7. c	20. d	33. b	46. c	59. a
8. d	21. a	34. c	47. c	60. b
9. a	22. b	35. a	48. b	61. c
10. d	23. d	36. b	49. b	62. b
11. b	24. b	37. b	50. c	63. a
12. b	25. b	38. d	51. c	64. d
13. c	26. b	39. b	52. b	65. a

CHAPTER 15—HAIRSTYLING

1. b	12. c	23. b	34. c	45. a
2. c	13. b	24. a	35. c	46. a
3. b	14. a	25. d	36. b	47. a
4. c	15. d	26. a	37. c	48. b
5. b	16. a	27. b	38. b	49. a
6. d	17. c	28. b	39. b	50. b
7. a	18. b	29. c	40. a	51. a
8. b	19. a	30. a	41. a	52. a
9. d	20. b	31. d	42. c	53. b
10. a	21. c	32. b	43. d	54. a
11. a	22. d	33. a	44. a	55. d

CHAPTER 16—BRAIDING AND BRAID EXTENSIONS

1. b	7. d	13. a	19. a	25. d
2. b	8. b	14. a	20. c	26. a
3. a	9. d	15. d	21. b	27. d
4. d	10. b	16. b	22. a	28. d
5. c	11. a	17. a	23. b	29. b
6. b	12. a	18. b	24. b	30. a

CHAPTER 17—WIGS AND HAIR ENHANCEMENTS

1. b	7. b	13. d	19. c	25. a
2. b	8. d	14. b	20. d	26. d
3. c	9. b	15. a	21. a	27. a
4. a	10. a	16. b	22. b	28. d
5. c	11. c	17. b	23. a	29. c
6. d	12. c	18. d	24. d	30. a

CHAPTER 18—CHEMICAL TEXTURE SERVICES

1. b	14. b	27. a	40. a	53. d
2. d	15. d	28. b	41. a	54. b
3. a	16. a	29. b	42. b	55. b
4. b	17. b	30. a	43. d	56. c
5. a	18. c	31. d	44. b	57. a
6. b	19. d	32. b	45. a	58. a
7. b	20. a	33. c	46. b	59. c
8. d	21. b	34. b	47. a	60. b
9. b	22. a	35. a	48. c	61. c
10. a	23. d	36. b	49. b	62. b
11. c	24. a	37. d	50. b	63. c
12. b	25. b	38. c	51. b	64. d
13. a	26. c	39. a	52. b	65. c

CHAPTER 19—HAIRCOLORING

1. b	15. b	29. c	43. c	57. b
2. a	16. b	30. b	44. b	58. a
3. d	17. d	31. d	45. d	59. b
4. a	18. b	32. c	46. c	60. b
5. a	19. b	33. a	47. c	61. d
6. c	20. d	34. c	48. c	62. b
7. a	21. a	35. b	49. b	64. d
8. b	22. b	36. d	50. d	65. b
9. c	23. c	37. b	51. b	65. d
10. d	24. d	38. a	52. d	66. d
11. a	25. c	39. c	53. a	67. b
12. b	26. d	40. b	54. c	68. d
13. d	27. a	41. b	55. b	69. b
14. b	28. b	42. a	56. c	70. c

CHAPTER 20—SKIN DISEASES AND DISORDERS

1. b	7. d	13. a	19. d	25. d
2. d	8. d	14. b	20. b	26. c
3. a	9. b	15. c	21. a	27. b
4. b	10. d	16. b	22. c	28. d
5. c	11. a	17. b	23. b	29. b
6. b	12. d	18. a	24. a	30. a

CHAPTER 21—HAIR REMOVAL

1. b	6. a	11. a	16. d	21. d
2. c	7. a	12. d	17. a	22. b
3. a	8. b	13. d	18. b	23. a
4. d	9. b	14. c	19. c	24. a
5. b	10. d	15. b	20. b	25. b

CHAPTER 22—FACIALS

1. b	11. b	21. b	31. b	41. b
2. d	12. b	22. a	32. d	42. c
3. c	13. d	23. d	33. c	43. b
4. a	14. a	24. c	34. b	44. d
5. b	15. d	25. a	35. a	45. a
6. c	16. c	26. b	36. c	46. c
7. a	17. c	27. a	37. d	47. b
8. d	18. b	28. b	38. a	48. a
9. b	19. b	29. d	39. b	49. d
10. c	20. a	30. c	40. c	50. c

CHAPTER 23—FACIAL MAKEUP

1. c	7. c	13. c	19. a	25. c
2. d	8. b	14. b	20. b	26. a
3. a	9. a	15. c	21. b	27. c
4. a	10. c	16. d	22. b	28. b
5. b	11. d	17. c	23. d	29. b
6. b	12. b	18. a	24. a	30. b

CHAPTER 24—NAIL DISEASES AND DISORDERS

1. a	6. d	11. c	16. a
2. a	7. c	12. c	17. a
3. b	8. d	13. a	18. b
4. c	9. a	14. b	19. a
5. b	10. a	15. a	20. b

CHAPTER 25—MANICURING

1. b	8. c	15. d	22. d	29. c
2. c	9. b	16. a	23. a	30. b
3. b	10. d	17. a	24. c	31. a
4. d	11. c	18. c	25. b	32. a
5. b	12. c	19. b	26. c	33. d
6. b	13. b	20. c	27. a	34. a
7. a	14. b	21. d	28. b	35. c

CHAPTER 26—PEDICURING

1. b	6. a	11. b	16. d	21. a
2. c	7. d	12. a	17. a	22. b
3. b	8. b	13. b	18. d	23. c
4. d	9. c	14. c	19. c	24. b
5. c	10. b	15. b	20. b	25. d

CHAPTER 27—NAIL TIPS, WRAPS, AND NO-LIGHT GELS

1. b	6. a	11. d	16. b
2. a	7. b	12. c	17. d
3. d	8. d	13. d	18. d
4. b	9. c	14. b	19. d
5. c	10. a	15. c	20. b

CHAPTER 28—ACRYLIC (METHACRYLATE) NAILS

1. b	7. b	13. b	19. d	25. c
2. d	8. a	14. d	20. b	26. c
3. a	9. c	15. c	21. c	27. c
4. d	10. b	16. a	22. d	28. c
5. b	11. d	17. a	23. d	29. b
6. c	12. d	18. a	24. b	30. d

CHAPTER 29—UV GELS

1. b	6. b	11. b	16. b
2. c	7. d	12. a	17. b
3. c	8. c	13. c	18. a
4. b	9. b	14. b	19. c
5. d	10. c	15. a	20. b

CHAPTER 30—SEEKING EMPLOYMENT

1. b	6. b	11. a	16. b
2. c	7. d	12. a	17. a
3. d	8. a	13. d	18. b
4. d	9. d	14. c	19. a
5. a	10. b	15. a	20. d

CHAPTER 31—ON THE JOB

1. b	6. d	11. b	16. d
2. c	7. c	12. a	17. c
3. a	8. a	13. c	18. b
4. c	9. d	14. b	19. d
5. b	10. a	15. b	20. c

CHAPTER 32—THE SALON BUSINESS

1. b	6. a	11. c	16. d
2. a	7. c	12. a	17. c
3. c	8. c	13. b	18. a
4. b	9. a	14. c	19. d
5. d	10. b	15. a	20. b

NOTES